Cook Smart, Eat Well

MAYO CLINIC | Mayo Cli...

MAYO CLINIC

Author | Jennifer A. Welper
Publisher | Daniel J. Harke
Editor in Chief | Nina E. Wiener
Senior Editor | Karen R. Wallevand
Managing Editor | Anna L. Cavallo
Art Director | Stewart J. Koski
Production Design | Amanda J. Knapp
Photography | Michael T. Burrows, Paul Flessland, Matthew C. Meyer
Copy Editors | Miranda M. Attlesey, Alison K. Baker, Nancy J. Jacoby, Julie M. Maas
Indexer | Carol Roberts
Contributors | Jason S. Ewoldt, M.S., RDN; Laura M. Waxman
Image Credits | All photographs and illustrations are copyright of MFMER, except for the following: PAGE 13/ CREDIT: Sheri Giblin, Nancy R. Cohen

Published by Mayo Clinic Press

© 2022 Mayo Foundation for Medical Education and Research (MFMER)

The information in this book is true and complete to the best of our knowledge. This book is intended only as an informative guide for those wishing to learn more about health issues. It is not intended to replace, countermand or conflict with advice given to you by your own physician. The ultimate decision concerning your care should be made between you and your doctor. Information in this book is offered with no guarantees. The author and publisher disclaim all liability in connection with the use of this book.

For bulk sales to employers, member groups and health-related companies, contact Mayo Clinic, 200 First St. SW, Rochester, MN 55905, or email SpecialSalesMayoBooks@mayo.edu.

ISBN 978-1-893005-80-8

Library of Congress Control Number: 2021943835

Printed in the United States of America

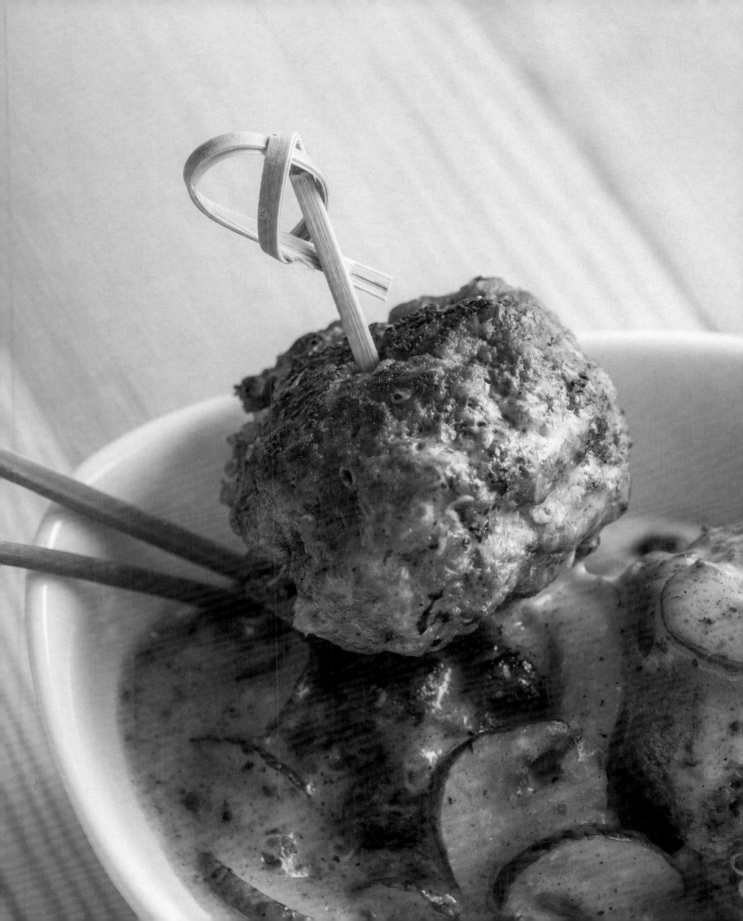

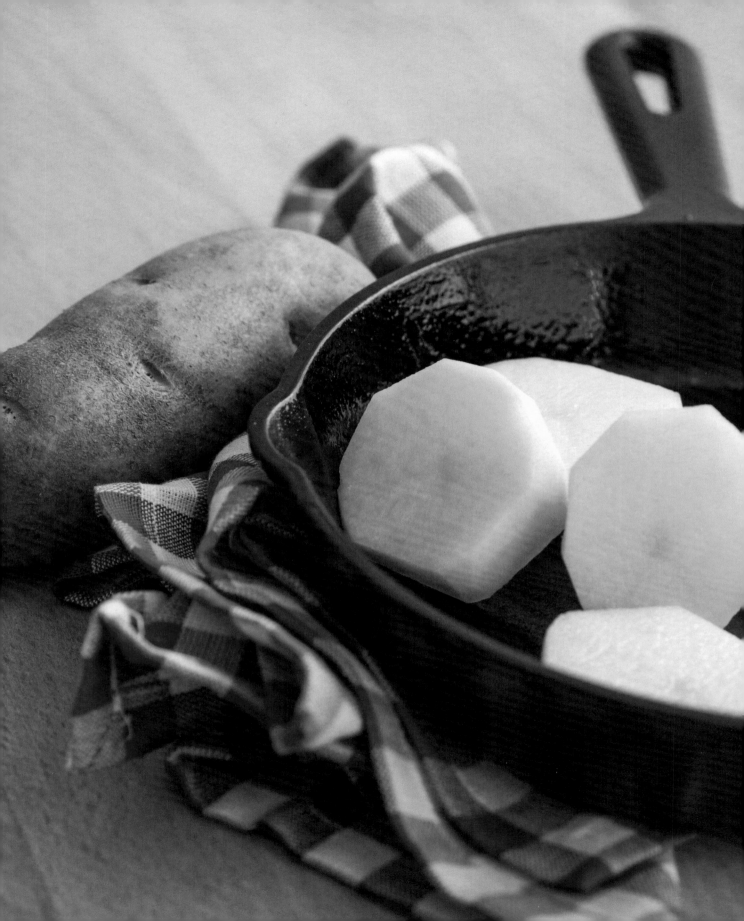

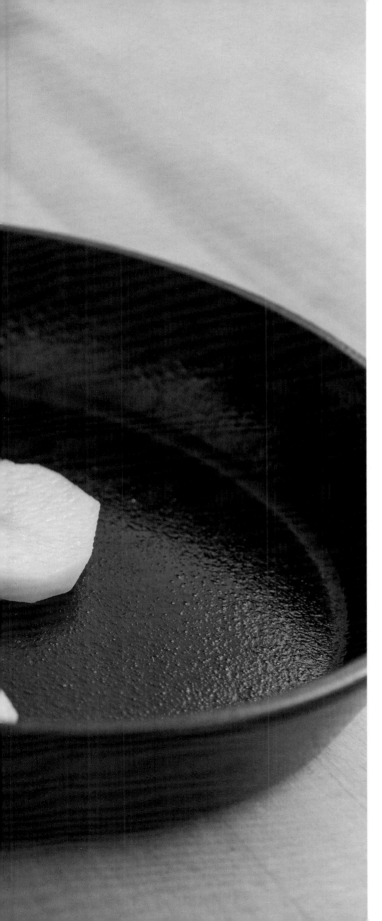

Contents

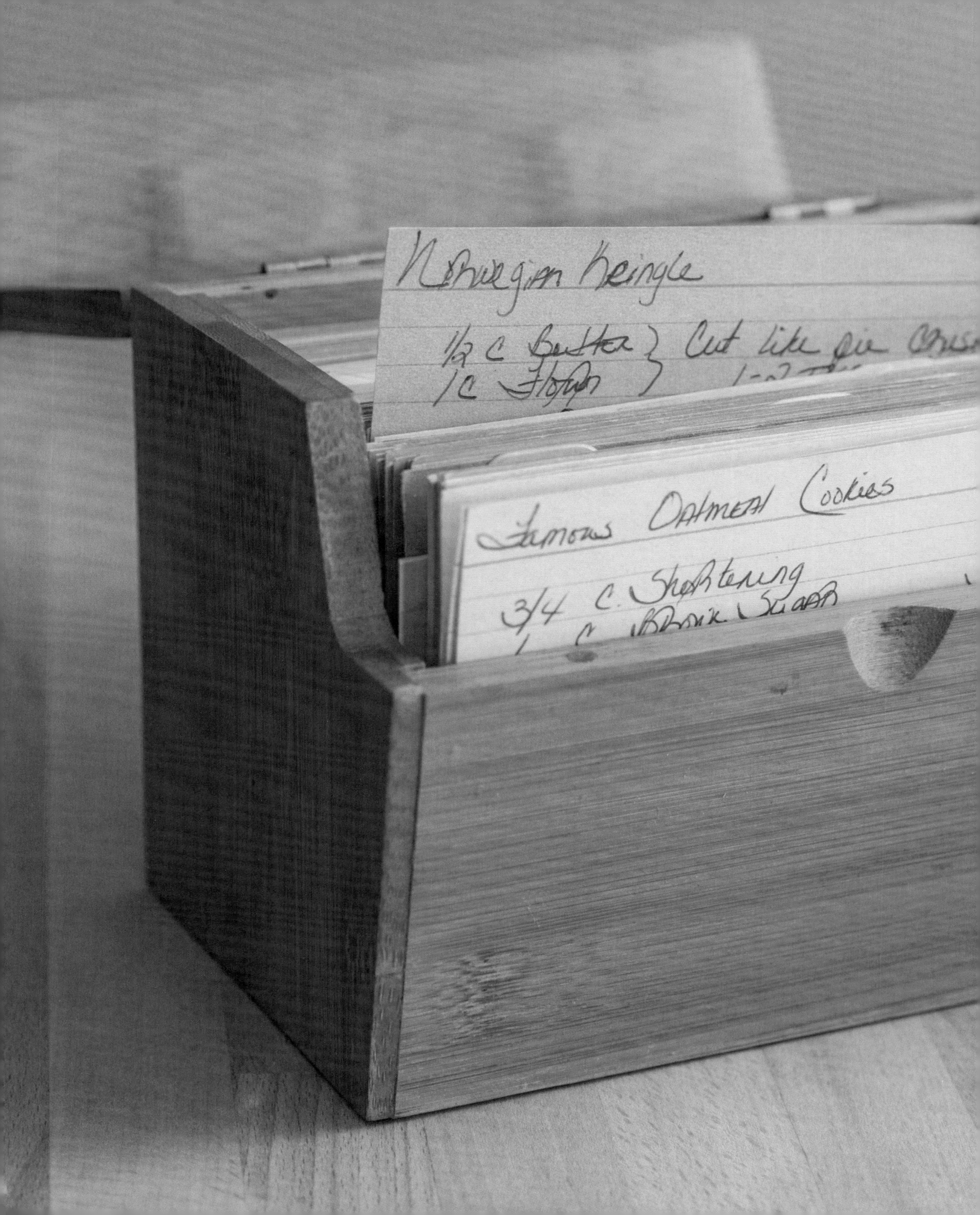

Norwegian Kringle

1/2 c Butter } Cut like pie crust
1 c Flour   } 1-2 Tbsp

Famous Oatmeal Cookies

3/4 c. Shortening
1 c. Brown Sugar

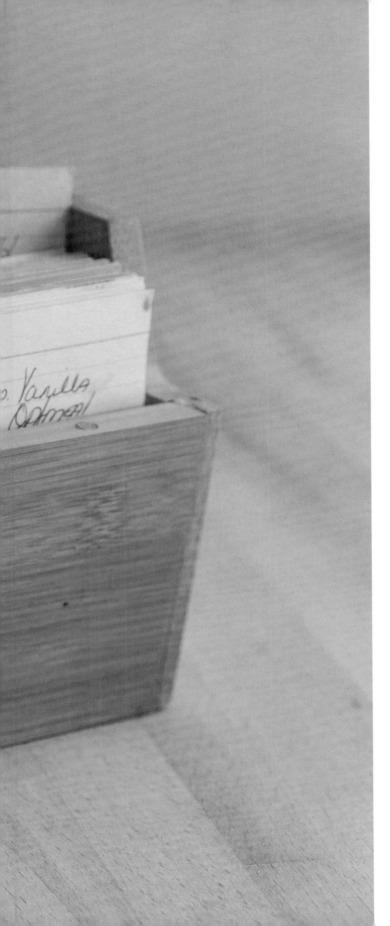

This book is dedicated to my mom, Colleen Welper, who passed away January 4, 2019.

She instilled in me at a young age the importance of health and the power of hospitality. She also passed on to me her drive and strong will. Without all of these gifts, this cookbook wouldn't be possible.

The recipe box pictured here is my mom's. A keepsake I treasure greatly!

May this cookbook be the foundation for many meals and memories to be shared — from my kitchen to yours, one recipe at a time.

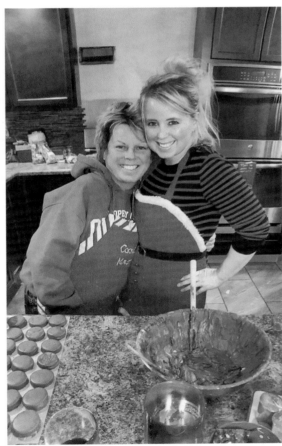

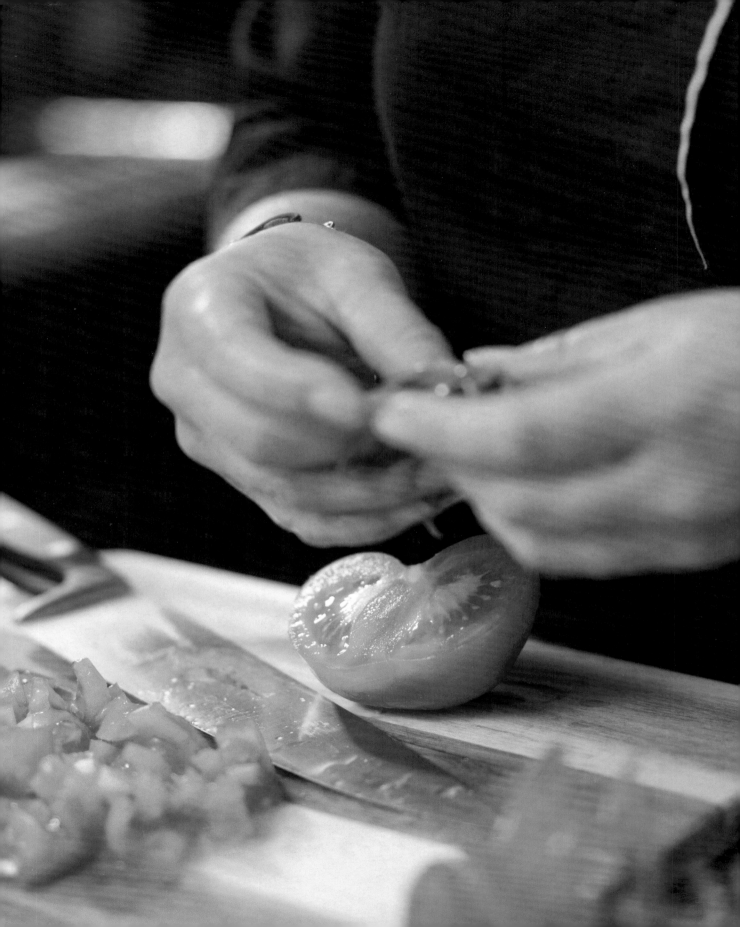

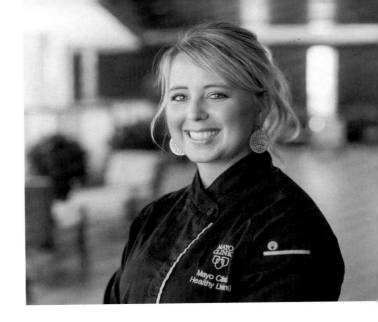

Introduction

Growing up on a dairy farm in southeastern Minnesota, I found my niche in the kitchen. I spent a lot of time alongside my mom and my grandmother who cooked traditional meat and potatoes meals for my large extended family. My mom was health conscious and aware of portion sizes, but hearty Midwestern meals were still pretty standard in our home. Before I left for culinary school, my grandfather died suddenly. He had struggled with diabetes, heart disease and controlling his weight. This loss infused me with a new passion. I wanted to learn how to make food that not only tasted good but was healthy and relatable — food my grandpa would have enjoyed!

My culinary journey eventually brought me to Mayo Clinic, where I am able to both cook and teach! In my classes, I've heard from many people with a range of cooking skills and an array of dieting experiences. From these interactions, I understand the struggles and frustrations people often have when it comes to cooking and eating healthy. It's with their stories in mind that I developed many of the recipes in this cookbook. My goal was to create a book that provides a solid foundation to healthy cooking and eating, with basic recipes, simple ingredients and timesavings tips.

As you dig in, make sure to look at the first two sections. They provide important resources on kitchen supplies, meal prep, cooking techniques and cross-utilization of ingredients. This information can help you better understand the why, when and how to be successful. For example, while the recipes in this book don't use heavy amounts of olive oil or butter, you can still achieve the same taste and appearance as dishes containing more fat by cooking the oil or butter at a lower temperature for a longer period of time. By paying close attention to these basic cooking techniques, you can prepare restaurant-quality meals without the calories.

It's my hope that the recipes in this cookbook will provide you with a new perspective on how to prepare easy meals that taste good and are good for you. I also hope that the cooking methods outlined in this book will help you master basic techniques of food preparation, which you can implement with your other favorite meals.

If you want to eat healthy without taking the *goodness* out of good food, look no further. Here's how to cook smart and eat well!

Jennifer A. Welper, Wellness Executive Chef

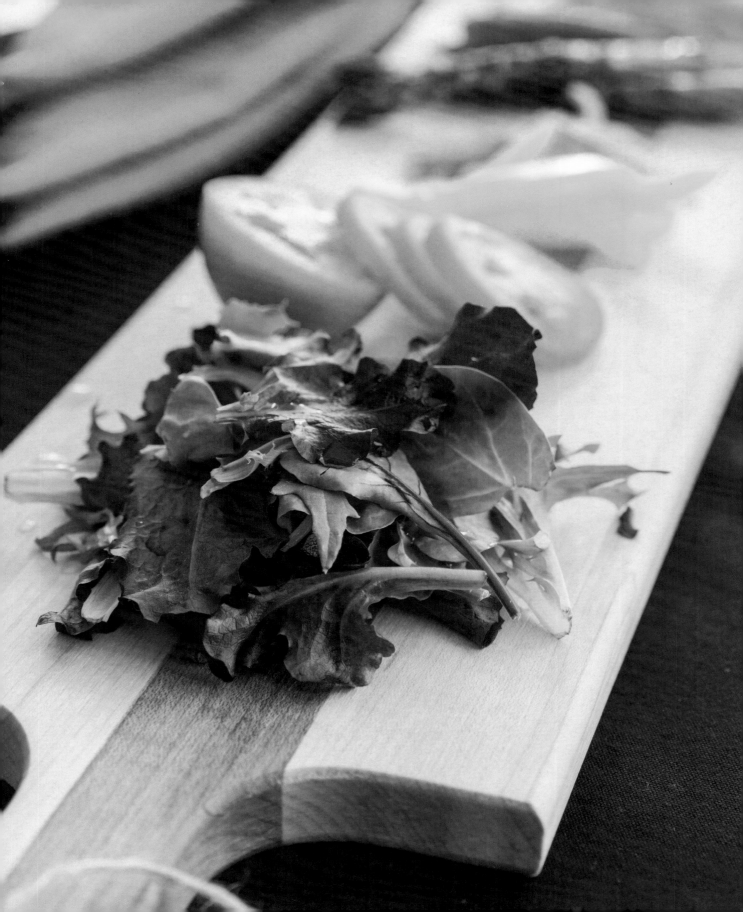

Foreword

Chances are, you probably know that your health is dictated to a great extent by your lifestyle habits, including your diet. The food you eat each day and the nutrients that food provides are important to your overall health and weight.

Research shows that a diet that includes plenty of vegetables, fruits, whole grains, nuts, beans and healthy fats such as olive oil — what's often referred to as a plant-based diet — can decrease your risk of heart disease and cancer and reduce your overall risk of death. Let me repeat that: Eating the right foods can help you avoid many diseases and live longer. Who doesn't want that?

In addition to your health, another reason you may be interested in this cookbook is because you've found that food affects how you feel — when you eat well, you feel well! Nutritious meals not only give you more energy but also stimulate your mood. When you eat well, you feel good knowing that you're fueling your body with healthy nutrients rather than unhealthy foods.

Plus, food brings people together. We enjoy sharing our favorite foods. Whether it's a holiday celebration, a weekday meal with family or a caring basket for a friend or neighbor, food can warm our hearts as well as our stomachs. Exploring new healthy recipes adds to this enjoyment.

Yet another reason you might be attracted to this cookbook may be the most important — you're looking for easy and appealing recipes to motivate you to action. How many times have you thought, "I need to eat better" or "I should learn how to cook healthier." Most people know what they need to do, they just have trouble actually doing it! Here's your chance to learn to do something really important for yourself and your family.

Cook Smart, Eat Well is about eating better without having to invest a lot of time. If you're worried a healthy diet means a boring and bland diet, think again! There's no reason that nutritious foods that are easy to prepare can't be tasty and enjoyable. Chef Jennifer Welper combines practical cooking tips with simple yet great-tasting recipes to show you how approachable and satisfying healthy eating can be.

Here's to a healthier and happier you!

Donald D. Hensrud, M.D., M.P.H., General Internal Medicine, Mayo Clinic; Associate Professor of Nutrition and Preventive Medicine, Mayo Clinic College of Medicine and Science

Eating to the pyramid

Below the title of each recipe in this cookbook you'll find some colorful dots. These dots provide information that can help you eat a healthier diet that includes a balance of foods and nutrients.

The recipes in this cookbook are based on the overall philosophy of the Mayo Clinic Healthy Weight Pyramid, shown on the opposite page. The pyramid was developed based on research that suggests a diet that's primarily plant-based is the healthiest.

Following a plant-based diet doesn't mean that you need to adopt a vegetarian or vegan lifestyle in order to live healthy. Rather, it means that fruits and vegetables should make up the foundation of your daily meals. These are the foods that you want to eat the most of.

Use the pyramid as a guide for making smart dietary choices to help you eat well and benefit from key nutrients found in different foods. Adhering to the core concepts of the pyramid also is an effective way to lose weight if that's one of your overall goals.

Moving up the pyramid, you'll find additional food groups that are important to a healthy diet beyond fruits and vegetables. When eating carbohydrates, make sure to select whole-grain products such as whole-grain pasta and whole-wheat bread. They're better choices than their refined counterparts. When purchasing protein and dairy products, choose mainly lean or low-fat options. These include foods such as fish, lean poultry, beans and skim milk.

Some fat is important to a healthy diet but you want to include foods that contain heart-healthy unsaturated fats, such as nuts and olive oil. Finally, an occasional sweet is OK, but it shouldn't be part of every meal.

To put the pyramid into action, there's a certain mix of food groups that you want to aim for each day. The number of servings to target depends on your weight and whether you're trying to lose weight or maintain a healthy weight. For example, for a woman who weighs 250 pounds or less and is trying to lose some weight, her daily target would be to eat at least 4 servings of vegetables, at least 3 servings of fruits, along with 4 servings of carbohydrates, 3 servings of protein/dairy and 3 servings of fats.

You can learn more about the Mayo Clinic Healthy Weight Pyramid, including information on the different target levels and how many servings of each food group to eat to reach your daily target at *diet.MayoClinic.org*.

For this cookbook, the dots below each recipe title let you know what food groups and how many servings from each of those food groups are found in one recipe serving.

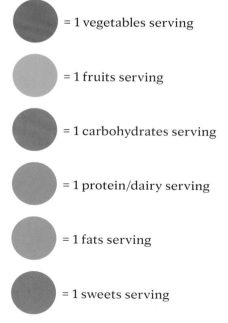

= 1 vegetables serving

= 1 fruits serving

= 1 carbohydrates serving

= 1 protein/dairy serving

= 1 fats serving

= 1 sweets serving

Mayo Clinic Healthy Weight Pyramid

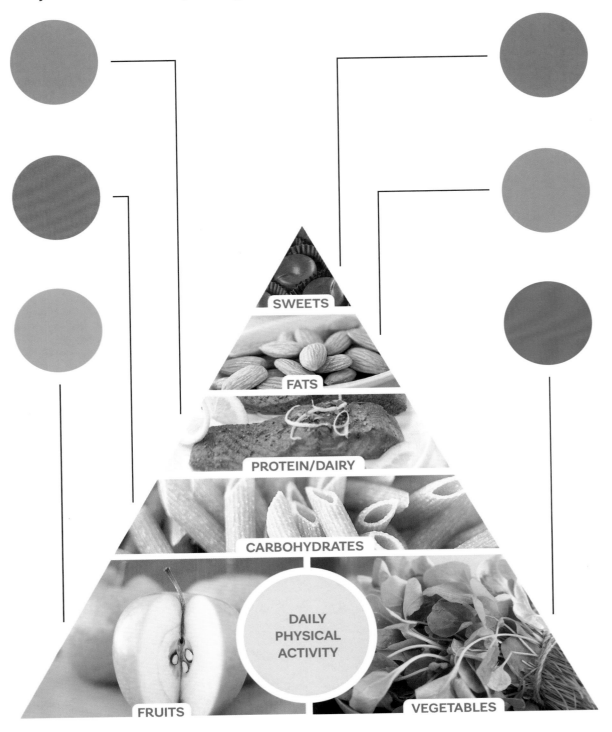

SWEETS

FATS

PROTEIN/DAIRY

CARBOHYDRATES

DAILY PHYSICAL ACTIVITY

FRUITS

VEGETABLES

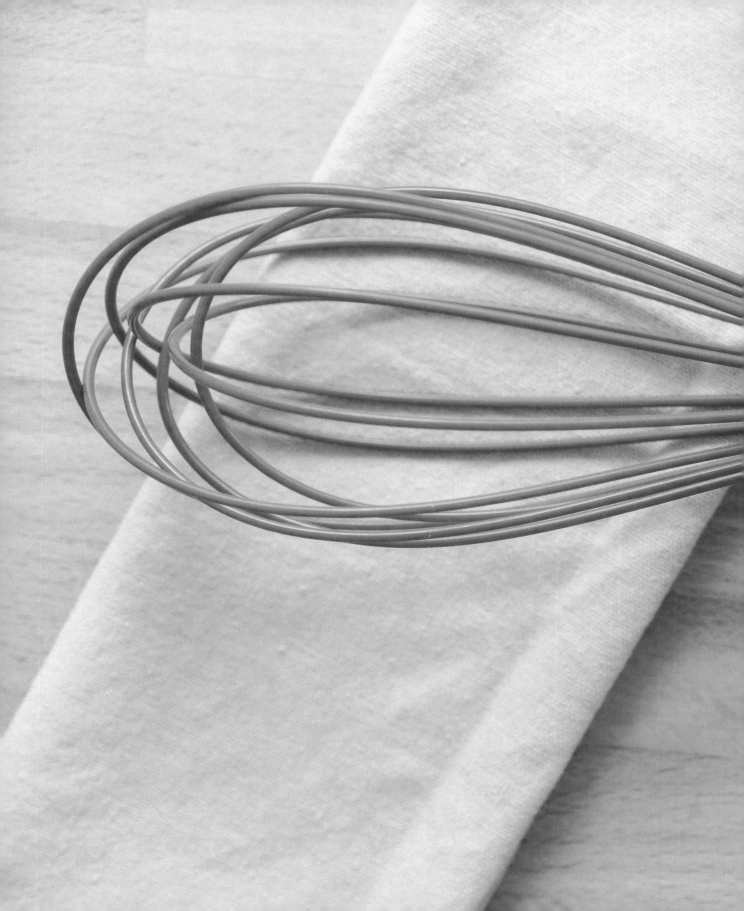

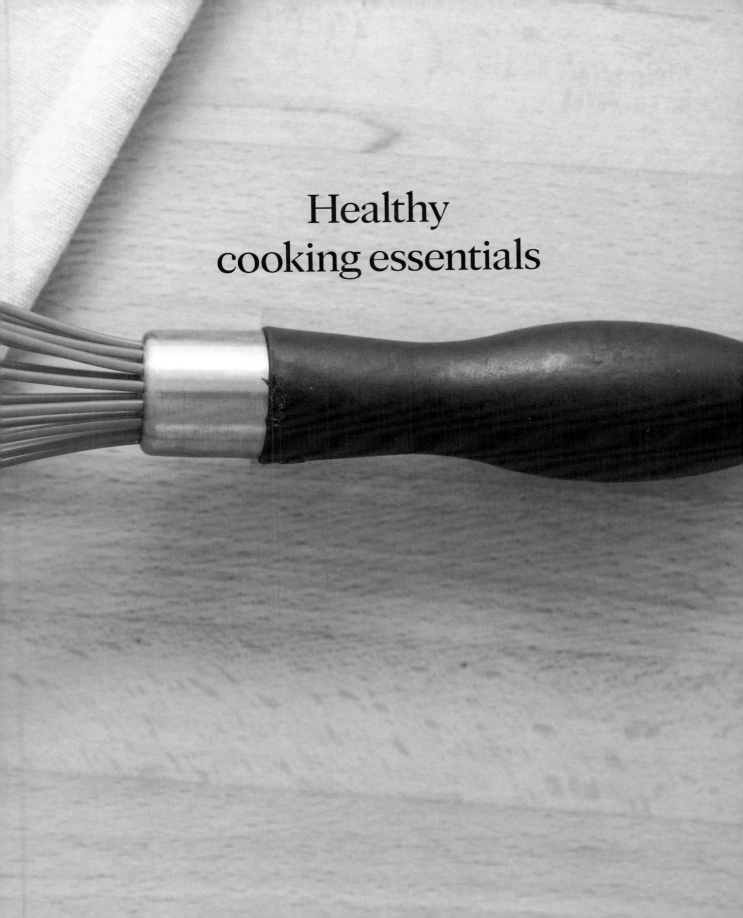

Healthy cooking essentials

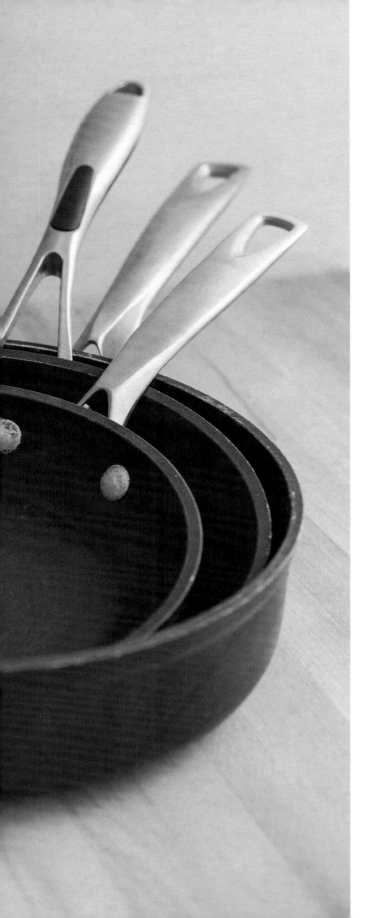

Healthy, flavorful meals are well within reach for anyone. Really! This book is full of recipes that you can put together relatively quickly with basic cooking techniques. But before you dig into the pages ahead, make sure you set yourself up for success with some simple tools and tricks of the trade.

Whether you're brand new to cooking or have been at it for a while, this chapter offers something for everyone. It'll walk you through basic equipment you'll want to have in your kitchen, along with ingredients it's always good to have on hand. You'll also read about different types of food preparation methods, in addition to tips that can help make meal prep a smooth, efficient and enjoyable experience.

These concepts are important because they empower you to step into your kitchen with confidence, so that you can prepare tasty, enjoyable and healthy meals for you and your family.

As you take steps to eat better, you'll probably be eating differently than you have in the past. You may find yourself purchasing more fruits and vegetables, more rice and whole-grain products, and more seafood and chicken than you're used to.

At first, all of these changes may seem daunting because you've been separated from your normal routine. Try to be patient. With time, the process will get easier and gradually become second nature.

Remember, learning to cook healthy doesn't mean you have to become a gourmet chef or invest in all sorts of gadgets and tools. Just follow the standard cooking methods out-lined in this chapter, and make sure your kitchen is equipped with a few key items for food preparation. That's it!

Kitchen staples

To cook enjoyable meals throughout the week, you don't need fancy or expensive cookware. A core set of equipment is all you'll need for these recipes. Chances are, you already have a lot of these items in your kitchen. If you're missing some, don't worry. Many recipes can be made with the kitchen equipment you have on hand. And, of course, you can always add new equipment over time, as you're able.

Cookware

Most recipes rely on a small collection of cookware to get the job done. These are the items you'll be turning to again and again.

PANS | Aim to have two sizes of good-quality sauté pans or skillets in your kitchen. Non-stick pans, such as hard-anodized pans, are ideal for healthy cooking. Unlike stainless steel, nonstick surfaces allow you to cook with a small amount of oil so you don't need to add a lot of extra fat and calories just to cook your food.

A smaller pan is useful for scrambling eggs or searing a single piece of meat. A larger, deeper pan allows you to sear multiple pieces of meat, sauté large amounts of vegetables, or cook bulkier meals such as rice pilaf or pasta dishes.

POTS | You'll want a smaller pot for preparing sauces, such as homemade teriyaki or barbecue sauce. Use a larger pot for making soups or big batches of pasta or rice.

BAKING SHEETS | Stock your kitchen with at least one good-quality baking sheet for roasting vegetables and cooking or roasting meats and other foods.

BAKING PAN | You'll want a 9x13 inch baking pan for dishes such as casseroles or for baking some meats and vegetables.

CAST IRON SKILLET GRILL | This item isn't necessary if you have access to an outdoor grill, but it can be a convenient option if you don't have a grill or prefer to grill indoors.

ROASTING OR BROILING PAN | If you plan to roast or broil meat often, these pans can aid in healthy cooking. Their racks allow fat to drip away from the meat while cooking.

Knives

You probably have a variety of knives in your kitchen. From small to large, each type of knife is designed for a specific purpose. The knife you'll be relying on most when preparing recipes is a chef's knife.

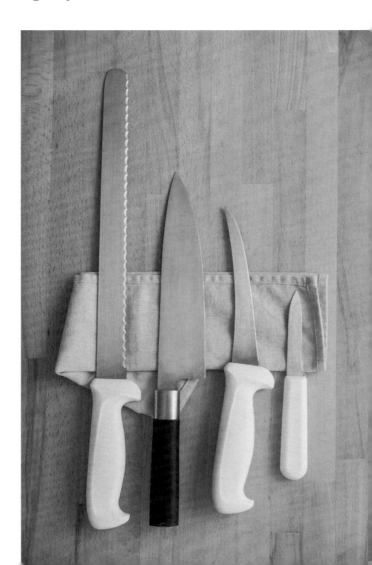

- CHEF'S KNIFE | With a broad blade that tapers down to a point, this knife is the workhorse of the kitchen. It can be used for most of your cutting needs, including slicing and chopping vegetables and meat.
- BREAD KNIFE | The job of this rectangular serrated knife is to cut through bread.
- PARING KNIFE | This small, pointed knife can be used to peel, slice and mince fruits and vegetables.
- UTILITY KNIFE | Slightly larger than a paring knife, a utility knife is another versatile knife. It can slice vegetables and small breads, such as bagels.

CHOOSING AND CARING FOR YOUR CHEF'S KNIFE

There are several types of chef's knives. The one that's best for you comes down to personal preference. Some people prefer a heavier Western-style chef's knife with a hefty handle, while others like something more lightweight, such as a Japanese-style santoku knife.

What matters is that you keep your knife sharp. A sharp knife slices cleanly through food, making cutting and chopping more efficient and effortless. If you find yourself switching to a serrated knife to get the job done, it probably means your chef's knife has become too dull.

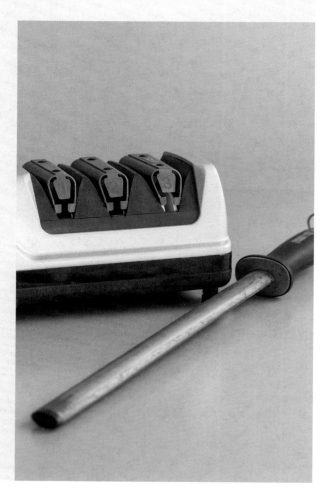

There are two ways to keep your chef's knife sharp:

1. **Honing.** *This method uses a metal rod called a honing steel to hone, or straighten, the edge of a slightly dull blade. Honing involves sweeping each side of a knife's edge repeatedly along the honing steel. Honing a knife regularly can reduce the number of times it needs to be sharpened.*
2. **Sharpening.** *While honing straightens the edge of a knife's blade, sharpening grinds off a little of the edge to sharpen it. Even a regularly honed knife will get dull over time and need to be sharpened. Many kitchen supply or hardware stores will sharpen your knives professionally for a fee. You can also purchase a knife sharpener for home use.*

Other tools

Along with good cookware and a sharp knife, having some good-quality, basic kitchen tools at your fingertips will make meal preparation a breeze.

SPATULA | Stock your kitchen with a good-quality spatula for turning and flipping food. If you're using nonstick pans, the spatula should have a silicone coating or be made with high-heat rubber. That way, it won't scratch the nonstick surface.

WHISK | A good-quality whisk is another go-to tool. Be sure to use one with a silicone or high-heat rubber coating if you're using nonstick cookware.

PEELER | A good-quality peeler, such as a Y peeler or metal peeler, can make meal prep go more quickly.

MEASURING TOOLS | Have on hand a set of good-quality measuring cups and measuring spoons made of plastic or stainless steel, as well as a liquid measuring cup made of glass or plastic. You can use these tools to measure not only ingredients for recipes but also servings of food onto your plate.

TONGS | A pair of tongs will allow you to flip meat and toss vegetables with ease. If you're using nonstick cookware, use tongs with a nonmetal tip.

STRAINER | Keep on hand a wire strainer. Choose one that can rest on top of the larger pot you use to cook rice or soup. This gives the tool a double purpose as both a strainer and a steamer. (See page 40 for how to steam food with a strainer.)

LARGE CUTTING BOARD | A cutting board with a large surface allows you to cut many vegetables at a time, without running out of space. Polyethylene plastic and wood are the best cutting surfaces because they won't damage your knife the way glass or ceramic can. Polyethylene is easiest to clean and maintain while wood may require a little more care and maintenance.

INSTANT-READ THERMOMETER | An instant-read thermometer can ensure that you're not over- or undercooking chicken, fish or other meat.

HONING STEEL | If you don't have a honing steel, consider purchasing one for your kitchen to keep your knives sharp.

GRATER | A grater with large holes cuts food into ribbons and strands. Small holes work well for creating fine particles, as in zesting.

STORAGE BAGS AND CONTAINERS | Stock your kitchen with sealable bags and containers with a tight seal in a variety of sizes to store portioned food for meals throughout the week. (See the next section for food storage tips.)

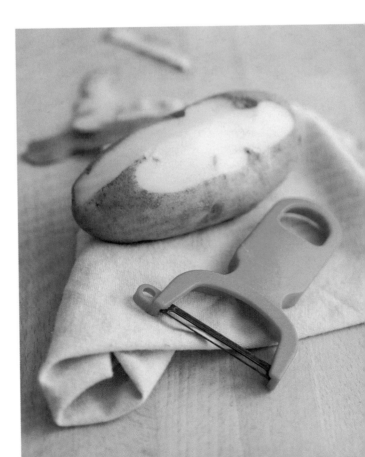

Core ingredients

The key to making healthy meals is having the right ingredients. After all, you can't eat — or prepare — what you don't have. To enjoy a nutritious, balanced diet, make sure that your kitchen is full of plenty of healthy options.

Shopping smart

Stocking your home with key ingredients begins at the grocery store. To maximize your time while shopping and cooking, be intentional and have a plan. Here are some basic strategies.

PLAN AHEAD | If you plan right, you should only need to grocery shop once or twice a week. Decide how many evening meals you'll be shopping for. Then consider food items you'll need for breakfasts, lunches and snacks. Take an inventory of essential foods in your house, such as fresh fruits and vegetables, whole grains, and low-fat dairy products.

As you plan, think about centering the week's meals around a manageable set of core ingredients rather than a wide selection of foods. (See pages 42-43 for a sample weekly meal plan). If you know you'll be purchasing peppers and onions for fajitas one night, buy some extra peppers and onions for pita pizzas another night. You'll cut down on the time spent shopping for different kinds of ingredients and preparing those ingredients.

MAKE A LIST | A list makes your shopping trip more efficient, and it helps you avoid impulse purchases. But don't let your list keep you from looking for or trying new food items. When making your list, use your meal plan for the week as your guide. Each recipe in this book includes those items you'll need to add to your grocery list and those to check for in your pantry or refrigerator. Make sure your list also includes healthy and convenient snacks.

READ NUTRITION LABELS | Check nutrition labels for serving size, calories, fat and sodium. Remember, even low-fat and fat-free foods can pack a lot of calories. Compare similar products so that you can choose healthier options.

Food staples

Healthy meals can come together in minutes — if you keep your kitchen stocked with some handy and healthy staples. When putting together your shopping list, make sure you're keeping your kitchen supplied with the following items:

Fruits and vegetables
- Fresh vegetables (including pre-cut, if desired)
- Frozen vegetables (no sauce)
- Salad in a bag
- Fresh fruits

FRESH VS. FROZEN VEGETABLES: WHICH TO CHOOSE?

Both fresh and frozen vegetables are good options for most recipes, and both pack healthy vitamins and fiber. Frozen vegetables have the advantage of being pre-cut and cooked, saving you time in the kitchen. But their taste and texture can be a little different from fresh vegetables.

Harder vegetables such as broccoli, carrots, corn and cauliflower tend to retain their texture better than softer vegetables, such as onions and peppers. But it's entirely up to you. Let your own preferences guide your decision to buy fresh or frozen.

SELECTING HEALTHY MEATS

To eat healthy, you want to buy the leanest cuts of meat. Lean meat options deliver flavor without containing a lot of marbled fat. You'll also be getting more bang for your buck, since lean meats contain more protein per pound than fattier meats. Look for these meats in the grocery store:

While these meat options are recommended for maintaining a healthy diet, that doesn't mean you can never eat other cuts of meat. If you plan to use a fattier meat on occasion, just try to plan the rest of your meal accordingly. Pair a small serving of the meat with a larger portion of vegetables, a flavorful whole-grain carbohydrate, a sprinkling of pungent cheese, or other filling and satisfying ingredients.

When it comes to cooking lean meats, keep in mind that they cook more quickly than fattier cuts of meat. While it's important to cook meat to a safe internal temperature, your meat will taste best if it's not overcooked. (See the chart on meat safety on the next page.) Lean meats tend to dry out and get tough when they're cooked for too long or at too high of heat, tempting you to add extra calories with more oils and sauces.

One way to prevent overcooking is to heat meat to about 5 degrees below the required minimum internal temperature. Then turn off the heat and let the meat rest for a few minutes before cutting or serving it. Its internal temperature will keep rising as the carryover heat within the meat continues to cook it. Before serving, check the meat again to ensure it has reached a safe temperature after resting. If not, reapply heat to finish cooking it.

TYPE OF MEAT	LEANEST OPTION	SECOND BEST OPTION
Poultry	Skinless chicken breast Ground turkey or chicken	Skinless dark meat (thigh)
Pork	Tenderloin	Loin
Beef	Tenderloin (filet mignon) 93% lean ground beef	Sirloin

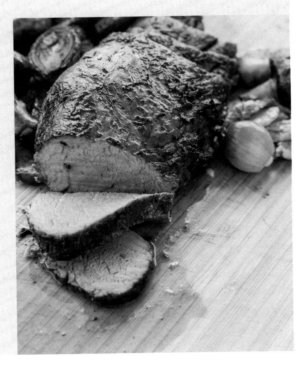

- Canned fruits (packed in their own juice or water)
- Frozen fruits

Whole grains
- Rice (brown, wild, blends)
- Oatmeal
- Whole-grain bread
- Whole-grain pita bread
- Whole-grain tortillas
- Whole-grain pasta
- Whole-grain breakfast cereal

Protein
- Low-fat refried beans
- Canned or dried beans (black, kidney or other favorites)

- Low-sodium water-packed tuna
- Other fish with omega-3s (fresh or frozen)
- Skinless white meat poultry
- Lean cuts of beef or pork
- Tofu
- Natural peanut butter

Dairy
- Low-fat or fat-free yogurt or Greek yogurt
- Lower fat or part-skim cheese
- Reduced-fat (Neufchatel) cream cheese
- Fat-free or 1% milk

Dairy alternatives, if desired
- Coconut or soy yogurt
- Soy, rice, oat or almond milk
- Dairy-free cheese

SAFE INTERNAL TEMPERATURES

Cooking meat to a safe internal temperature kills harmful organisms, preventing food poisoning. To correctly check the internal temperature of meat, insert an instant-read thermometer at an angle into the thickest part of the meat. Be sure the thermometer doesn't touch bone, fat or gristle.

Start checking the internal temperature when the meat is close to done but not fully cooked. That way, you can make sure you're not overcooking it. If the meat is still below the minimum internal temperature, be sure to clean the thermometer with soapy water before reinserting it into the meat the next time you check.

TYPE OF FOOD	MINIMUM INTERNAL TEMP
Beef, pork, veal and lamb (ground)	160 F
Beef, pork, veal and lamb (steaks, roasts and chops)	145 F
Chicken or turkey (all forms)	165 F
Fish with fins	145 F
Other seafood (shrimp, lobster, crab and scallops)	Cook thoroughly until flesh is pearly or white and also opaque.

Sauces

- Low-salt canned tomato sauce or paste
- Low-salt soy or tamari sauce

Spices and blends

Just as variety is the spice of life, spices and herbs add variety to your food. They infuse meals with flavor without adding extra calories. You can rub spices and herbs on meat, seafood and plant-based proteins or toss them with vegetables. Keep this core set of spices on hand:

- Coarse kosher salt
- Ground black pepper
- Basil
- Cayenne
- Chili powder
- Cinnamon
- Cumin
- Garlic
- Ginger
- Onion powder
- Oregano
- Paprika
- Red pepper flakes

Check out page 252 in the appendix for more guidance on spices and some suggestions for spice blends to add pizazz to your meals.

Oils

Canola and olive oils are some of your healthiest options when it comes to preparing vegetables, seafood, and meat or dressings for salads. To change up the flavor, try adding a small amount of savory oils to your dishes. Coconut oil and oils made from nuts and seeds — such as sesame and walnut oil — can add an extra dimension of flavor. Don't be afraid to experiment. Add a little to your pan, or sprinkle some on salads or cooked dishes.

Vinegars

Vinegar helps bring out flavor and depth. A splash of vinegar can enhance dressings, marinades, sauces, fresh vegetables and cooked dishes. Options to try include balsamic, wine or rice vinegar.

Sugar

Used sparingly, sugar can help thicken cooked marinades and sauces and add a caramelized flavor. If you need to limit or avoid sugar due to a health condition, you can often leave out the sugar or replace it with a sugar substitute. Just be aware that sugar substitutes will produce a slightly different flavor and may not thicken or caramelize the way sugar does.

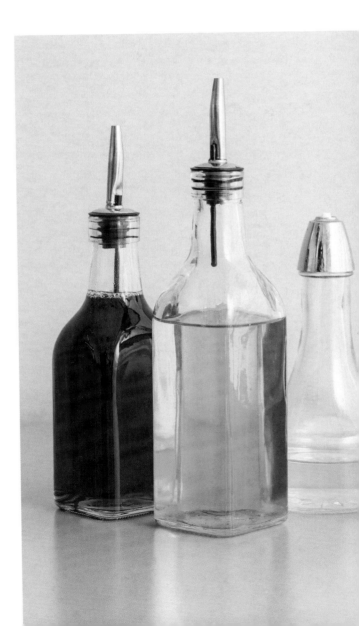

Preparing meals

Being successful in the kitchen doesn't mean you have to suddenly become a gourmet chef. Standard food preparation methods and cooking techniques can help you prepare a wide variety of meals that are as tasty as they are healthy. The following tips can help turn even beginners into efficient, confident cooks.

Cutting fresh vegetables

Along with fruits, vegetables are the foundation of a healthy diet. But if you're daunted by the idea of chopping up a mountain of veggies for a recipe, you're not alone. This step of the food preparation process can seem like a chore, but it doesn't have to be. Use these cutting methods to make all that slicing and dicing go surprisingly fast. A chef's knife is all you'll need.

BELL PEPPERS | Many people use a paring knife to carve the seeds out of a pepper before slicing it. However, using a chef's knife can be a quicker and easier method if you follow these steps.

1. Cut off the four sides, bottom and top of the pepper. Stand the pepper on its bottom. Lift the chef's knife with your wrist and drive it down into one side of the pepper to slice off a slab. Repeat with the three remaining sides and bottom, being careful to avoid the cluster of seeds in the middle. Cut off the remaining flesh of the pepper around the stem. Discard the stem and seeds. Now, you can slice or dice the pepper.
2. Slice. Place one slab of the pepper skin-side down on the cutting board. (Cutting a pepper skin side up puts too much pressure on the pepper, causing it to bruise and lose moisture.) Use a back-and-forward technique to cut the pepper into slices.

3. Dice. Turn the sliced pepper a quarter turn and use a back-and-forward technique to dice the slices crosswise into squares.

ZUCCHINI | There are a couple ways to cut vegetables such as zucchini, depending on the shape you're looking for.

Sticks and cubes

1. Prepare the zucchini. With a chef's knife, cut off both ends of the zucchini. Cut the vegetable in half crosswise. This gives you two shorter cylindrical pieces that are easier to work with.
2. Cut planks. Stand one of the halves vertically on the cutting board. Cut the zucchini into several planks by slicing downward lengthwise.
3. Slice sticks. Stack the planks flat on the cutting board, cut side down. Use the back-and-forward technique to slice the planks lengthwise into sticks.
4. Chop into cubes. Turn the sticks a quarter turn. Use a back-and-forward technique to chop the sticks crosswise into cubes.

Half circles

1. To prepare the zucchini, follow step 1 above.
2. Cut halves. Stand one of the cylindrical halves vertically on the cutting board. Slice it lengthwise down the middle, cutting it in half.
3. Cut half circles. Lay one of the halves on the cutting board, cut side down. Use the back-and-forward technique to slice it crosswise into half circles.

ONIONS | Onions are found in many dishes, so you may frequently find yourself cutting onions. Onions can be used many different ways. Depending on the recipe you're preparing, there are a couple of ways to ready your onions.

USING A CHEF'S KNIFE

You'll get the most benefit from this handy knife if you know how to hold and use it. Here's how to gain the greatest power, control and efficiency from a chef's knife.

Hold the knife properly. *Rather than hold a chef's knife at the end of the handle, hold it close to the base of the blade. To achieve this position, wrap your middle, ring and pinky fingers around the handle. Point your pointer finger downward, resting it against the base of the blade and rest your thumb against the other side of the blade.*

Use your wrist. *Control the movement of your knife with your wrist rather than with your shoulder or upper arm.*

Position your body. *Stand close to the cutting surface so that you're positioned near the food you're cutting.*

Utilize a back-and-forward cutting technique. *Once your hand and body are well positioned, follow this cutting method for most of your slicing and dicing needs:*

1. *Rest the tip of the chef's knife on the cutting board, holding the handle up at an angle. The food you want to cut should be beneath the raised part of the blade.*
2. *Pulling your wrist back, drag the angled knife backward through the food.*
3. *Pushing down with your wrist, press the entire blade into the food and drive the knife forward to finish slicing.*

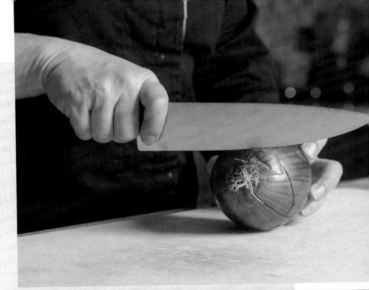

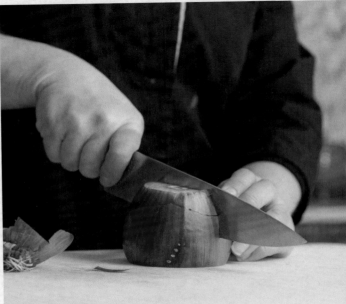

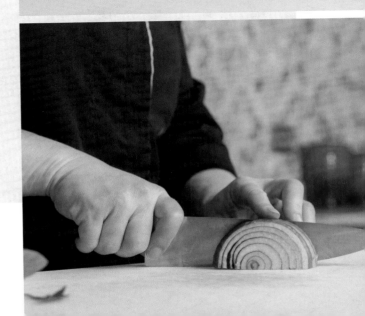

Slices and cubes

1. Prepare the onion. Cut off the ends. Stand the onion on one cut end and cut it in half down the middle, from end to end. Peel to remove the papery skin and the layer of tough waxy skin underneath.

2. Slice. Lay one half of the onion flat on a cutting board. Slice it crosswise, cutting in the same direction as the arcs within the onion. To do this, lift the knife over the onion and drive it down and forward. Pull the knife out, resting your pointer finger on the piece you just sliced to keep it in place. Repeat until the onion is sliced into half circles.

3. Dice if desired. Turn the sliced onion a quarter turn and tilt your knife at about a 45-degree angle, so the blade points in toward the center of the onion. Starting at one side of the onion, use the back-and-forward technique to cut across the slices at an angle. Gradually straighten out the knife with each new cut. When you get to the last quarter of the onion and it becomes hard to hold, tip it over so the side you just cut is now resting on the cutting board. Continue to chop the last quarter, beginning once again at an angle. Mincing is similar to dicing but uses a finer chop to create smaller cubes.

DETERMINING THE BEST SHAPE AND SIZE FOR CUT VEGGIES

When cutting a vegetable, a rule of thumb is to match the shape and size of the vegetable with the recipe you're making. This way, the vegetable will incorporate well into the dish, adding appealing color and texture and turning a modest portion of grain, pasta or protein into a sizable meal.

- **Small grains.** *If you're mixing vegetables with rice, quinoa or other small grains, cut thin slices and dice them — cutting again into small pieces.*
- **Shaped pasta.** *When mixing vegetables with shaped pasta, such as rotini or penne, cut them to roughly the same size as the pasta.*
- **Kebabs and roasted vegetables.** *Bigger vegetable chunks fit well on skewers and roast evenly on a baking sheet. Start by making thick slices and then chop the slices into squares.*
- **Stir-fries and fajitas.** *Thinner vegetable slices and julienned onions work well for these recipes.*

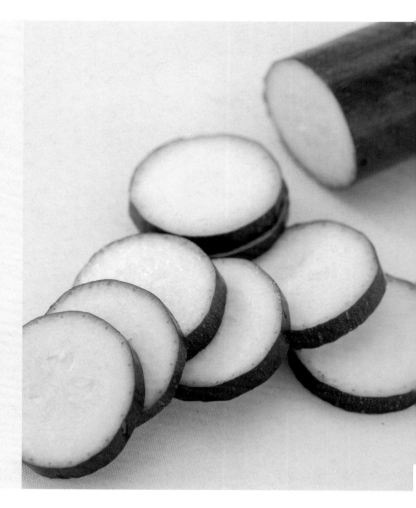

Julienned strips

1. Prepare the onion. Follow step 1 on the opposite page.
2. Julienne. Lay one half of the onion flat on the cutting board and slice it lengthwise, from end to end. Begin by tilting your knife at a 45-degree angle. Using the back-and-forward technique, cut thin strips. Gradually straighten the knife with each cut. Tip over the last quarter of the onion so that the side you just cut is now resting on the cutting board. Continue to chop the last quarter of the onion, beginning at an angle.

CARROTS | Similar to onions, carrots can be prepared in a variety of different ways. You can cut them into sticks for snacking. Some recipes call for carrots that are diced or cut in circles. If you're preparing stir-fries or perhaps a pasta dish, the recipe may suggest the carrots be sliced diagonally.

Sticks and cubes

1. Prepare the carrot. Peel the carrot to remove the skin. Cut off both ends. Cut the carrot crosswise into two cylindrical halves that are easier to manage.
2. Cut planks. Lay one carrot half on the cutting board with a cut end facing you. Anchor the chef's knife by resting its tip on the cutting board and inserting part of the blade into the far end of the carrot. Press the knife down fully into the carrot to slice off a plank. For thinner carrots, make this cut down the middle to create two planks. For thicker carrots, cut the carrot into three or four planks.
3. Cut sticks. Laying one plank cut side down, use the back-and-forward technique to slice it lengthwise into sticks.
4. Dice if desired. Turn the sticks a quarter turn. Dice them into squares by cutting crosswise using a back-and-forward technique.

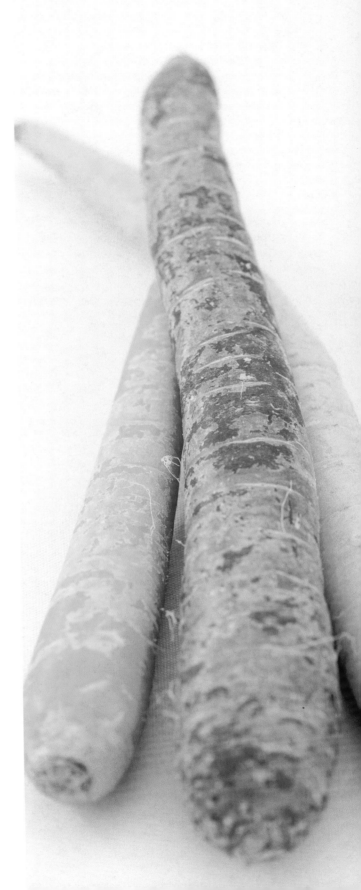

Diagonal slices
1. Follow steps 1 and 2 on the previous page.
2. Slice diagonally. Lay a plank cut side down. Slice the carrot lengthwise but at a diagonal to cut thin slices.

BREADING

Breading adds flavor and texture to baked meat by coating it with bread-crumbs. The simplest breading method is to sprinkle the breading on top of the meat before baking.

For a thicker breading, use this simple two-step process. First, dip the piece of meat in a shallow bowl containing whisked egg, letting any excess egg drip back into the bowl. Then dip the meat in a shallow bowl of breading, coating both sides. Place it on a baking sheet or pan to bake.

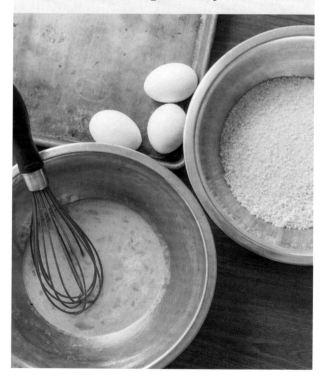

Cooking techniques

The recipes in this cookbook use a variety of simple cooking methods. These methods best capture the flavor and retain the nutrients in your food without adding too much fat or salt.

You'll notice that many of these methods call for preheating. A hot, preheated surface quickly cooks the outer layer of meats, plant-based proteins and vegetables, bringing out their natural flavor, aroma and appearance.

BAKING | Besides breads and desserts, you can bake seafood, poultry, lean meat, and vegetables and fruits that are somewhat uniform in size. Preheat the oven to the appropriate temperature. Place food in a pan or dish (covered or uncovered) and bake. If you're used to frying foods, baking or roasting is a good alternative.

GRILLING AND BROILING | Both grilling and broiling expose fairly thin pieces of food to direct heat and allow fat to drip away from the food. For grilling, use an outdoor grill or a cast iron skillet grill. For broiling, use a broiler rack below a heat element. Be sure to preheat the grill, skillet grill or broiler for a few minutes before adding any food.

When cooking pieces of meat or plant-based alternatives, avoid prodding or moving the food until it releases easily from the cooking surface. When broiling, cook the meat for the same amount of time on each side to cook it evenly. If you're grilling, cook the meat for a few minutes or until it releases easily. Then turn it a quarter turn on the same side and let it cook for another few minutes. Repeat on the other side. This helps the meat cook evenly and creates attractive crosshatch lines.

When grilling smaller items, such as vegetables, on an outdoor grill, place the food in a long-handled grill basket or on foil to prevent pieces from slipping through the rack.

ROASTING | Roasting uses an oven's dry heat at high temperatures to cook food placed on a baking sheet or in a roasting pan. Like baking, this is a good option if you're looking for a healthier alternative to frying. For poultry, seafood and meat, place a rack inside a roasting pan so that the fat can drip away during cooking.

When roasting vegetables, toss them in a small amount of oil or lightly mist a baking sheet with cooking spray to keep them from sticking to the pan. Lightly coating the vegetables with oil also helps them become crisp and browned. Spread the vegetables on the baking sheet so that they don't overlap. This will allow the oven's heat to circulate around them, cooking them evenly.

SAUTÉING | Sautéing cooks small or thin pieces of food in a shallow pan. Preheat the pan on high heat for a few minutes. To ensure the pan has reached a high enough temperature, flick a few droplets of water into the pan. If the water sizzles, the pan is ready to use.

Add a small amount of oil, cooking spray, low-sodium broth, water or wine, depending on the recipe. Add the food and stir it about every 30 seconds. When using less oil, sautéed food is likely to burn if cooked at high heat for too long, so you may need to turn down the heat to medium if you're used to recipes that call for more oil and higher heat. If you're still worried the food may burn on the outside before it's fully cooked, turn the heat down further or add a small amount of water to the pan and toss the food in it.

SEARING | Searing quickly browns the surface of food at a high temperature. It locks in flavor and moisture and adds an appealing golden crust to all types of meat, including poultry, fish and lean beef. Some plant-based proteins such as tofu and tempeh also can be seared.

Preheat a pan on medium heat for a few minutes until it's hot enough to make water droplets sizzle. Add a small amount of oil. Place the food in the pan for a few minutes or until the meat or protein releases easily from the pan. Flip it over to sear the other side.

After searing meat, finish cooking it to a safe internal temperature by turning down the heat and covering the pan. You can also transfer the meat to a baking pan or sheet and bake it in the oven.

STIR-FRYING | Stir-frying is similar to sautéing but cooks food more quickly. It works best with thin slices or small pieces of food that are uniform in size. Heat a large wok or pan on high heat until it's hot enough to make water droplets sizzle. Add a small amount of oil or cooking spray. Add the food, stirring it rapidly and continuously to prevent burning. To bring out the best flavor and texture in stir-fried vegetables, stir-fry them for a few minutes, or until the vegetables have turned a bright color and still retain some of their crispness.

STEAMING | One of the simplest cooking techniques to master is steaming food in a perforated basket, bamboo basket or wire strainer suspended above simmering liquid. Steaming can be used for a variety of vegetables, as well as tender meats such as fish and poultry. If you use a flavorful liquid or add herbs to the water, you'll flavor the food as it cooks. (See page 40 for a time-saving steaming tip.)

For meats, steam until the food has reached a safe internal temperature. Steam vegetables until they turn a bright color and retain some of their crispness.

If you're steaming a batch of vegetables for future meals, it's best to lightly blanch them. Steam them just until they begin to change color and then place them in a bowl of ice water to prevent further cooking.

Mix-and-match meals

It's easy when cooking to get caught in a rut. We tend to make the same things over and over again. This book includes more than 100 recipes that will show you how to pair basic ingredients in a variety of ways. Still, sometimes life calls for an even simpler approach. That's why it's helpful to experiment and learn how to improvise in ways that suit your tastes.

You don't need to purchase a lot of food or ingredients to mix and match your meals. Here are some ideas for how to combine different foods and ingredients to throw together an easy, satisfying meal or get out of a rut. Salads also can be an easy, filling meal to assemble in countless ways. Turn to page 80 for more ideas on mixing and matching salad ingredients for a tasty meal.

TRY 1 OF THESE PROTEINS	WITH 1 OF THESE SAUCES	PLUS 1 OF THESE CARBOHYDRATES	AND A LARGE PORTION OF VEGETABLES	
Beef tenderloin	BBQ	Brown rice	Asparagus	Green beans
Chicken breast	Hoisin	Brown rice pilaf	Bean sprouts	Lettuce
Ground lean beef	Marinara	Butternut squash	Beets	Mushrooms
Ground pork tenderloin	Marsala	Mashed or baked potatoes with the skin on	Bell peppers	Parsnips
Ground turkey breast	Teriyaki	Multigrain or whole-wheat pasta	Broccoli	Peas
Pork tenderloin		Oven-baked potato or sweet potato fries	Brussels sprouts	Snow peas
Tempeh			Cabbage	Spinach
Tofu (firm)		Quinoa	Carrots	Sugar snap peas
Turkey breast		Sweet potatoes with the skin on	Cauliflower	Summer squash

TRY 1 OF THESE SEAFOODS	WITH 1 OF THESE SAUCES			
Cod	Fat-free Italian dressing	Whole-wheat bread	Cucumbers	Turnips
Halibut	Lemon dill	Whole-wheat couscous	Eggplant	Zucchini
Salmon	Scampi	Whole-wheat tortillas		
Scallops	Sesame ginger			
Sea bass	Sweet and sour mango or pineapple salsa			
Shrimp	Teriyaki			
Tilapia	White wine			
Tuna				

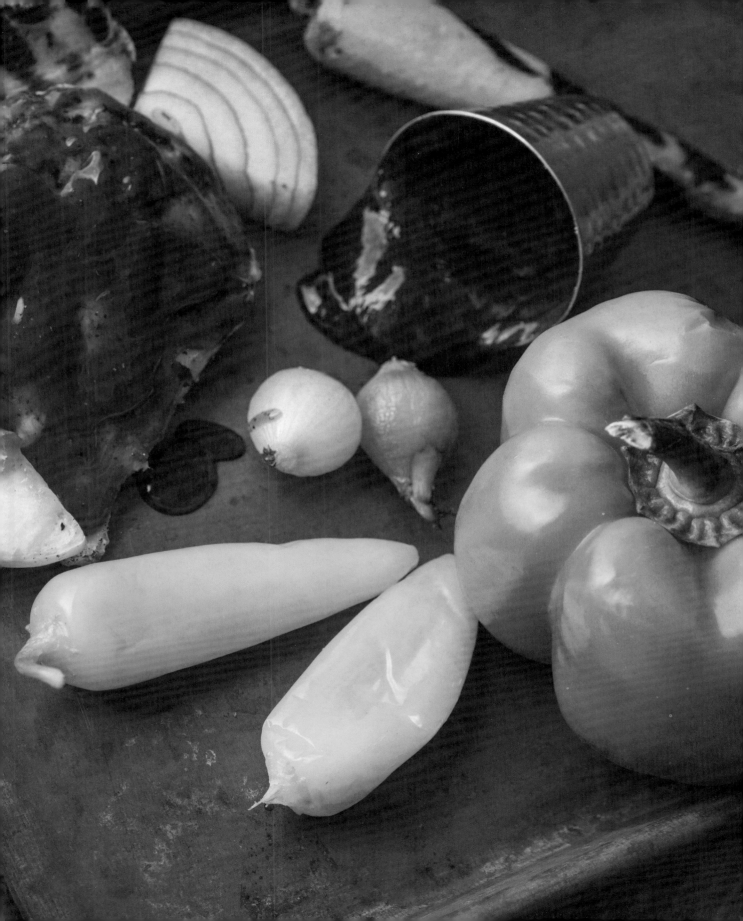

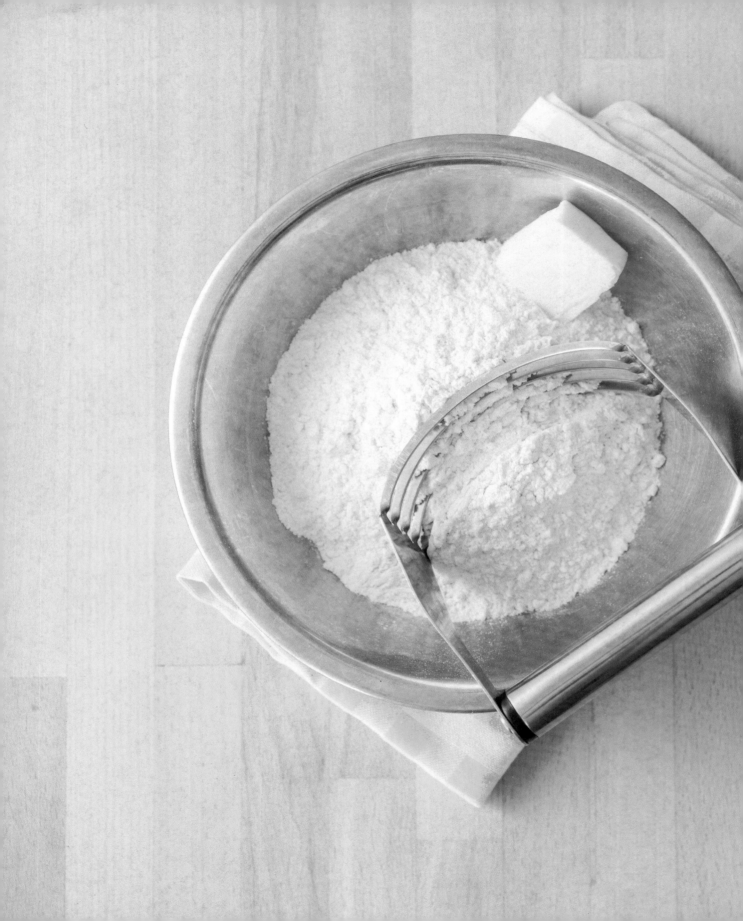

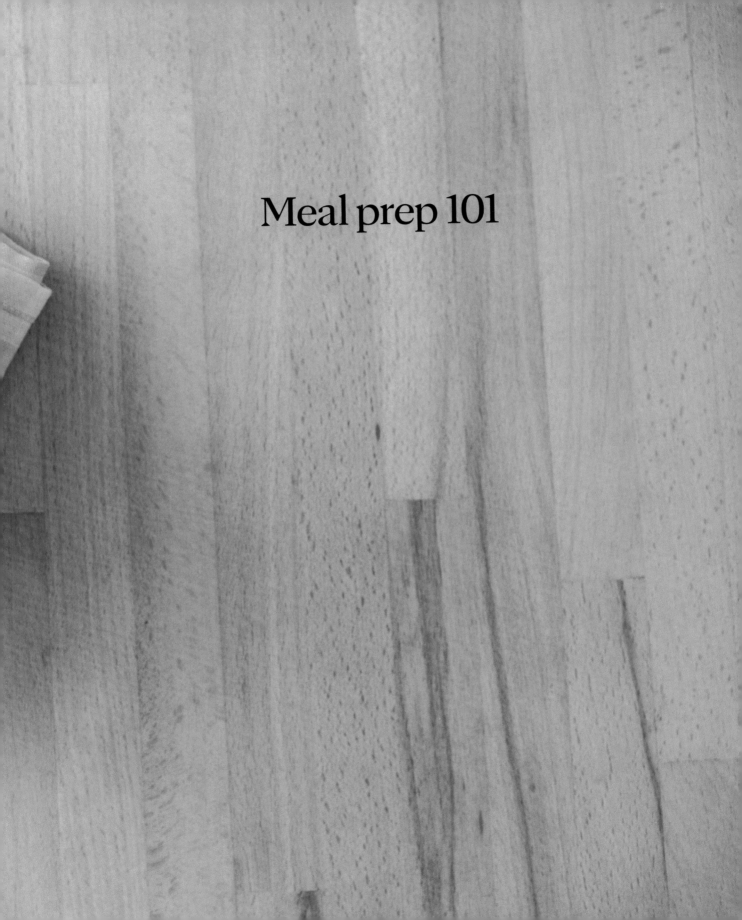

Meal prep 101

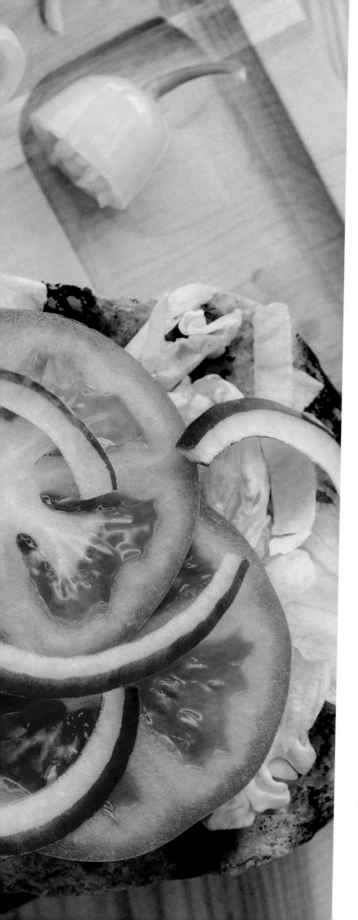

Preparing your own meals is good for your health. Making meals at home allows you to choose the ingredients that go into the food you eat, as well as control the portions being served. That's why eating at home is one of the best ways to maintain a balanced diet for yourself and your family. If you've purchased this cookbook, you probably already know most of this. But knowing and doing are often two different things!

Many people stop short when faced with the reality of continually preparing meals for themselves or their families. It can be hard enough sometimes to find the time or energy to make one meal, much less prepare an entire week's worth.

When it comes to cooking, it's important to have some type of weekly plan. If you don't have a plan, meal preparation becomes more difficult and time-consuming, which can make your cooking and eating experiences less enjoyable.

The recipes in this cookbook can help. They were created with busy people in mind. But timesaving recipes are only half the equation. Meal prep also is important.

The meal prep strategies outlined in this chapter will help you maximize your time and energy when you're working in the kitchen. They include simple tips for planning, preparing and assembling meals at home. For example, if you're cutting vegetables for today's soup, cut some more for tomorrow's pasta salad or a roasted vegetable sidedish later in the week.

The goal is to make these strategies part of your routine — part of your lifestyle — so that your inspiration to cook healthy is no longer a far-fetched fantasy but an attainable and practical reality.

Planning your week

The first step to being more efficient in the kitchen is meal planning. This involves charting out a week's menu ahead of time by organizing your meals around a manageable set of vegetables, grains and proteins. The suggestions that follow will help you put this timesaving strategy into practice.

Choose your ingredients

Focus your week's meal plan on four or five types of vegetables, three types of grain-based foods, and three proteins. These will be the core ingredients you'll use to compose your meals. When it's time to plan your menu for the next week, create some variety by swapping out one ingredient in each category and replacing it with something else.

The chart below shows you how three weeks of ingredients might look.

Cross-utilize your ingredients

Once you've decided on the ingredients you'll be working with for the week, look for ways to cross-utilize them. When you cross-utilize ingredients, you use them in a variety of combinations and with a variety of flavorings throughout the week. For example, If you're planning to use some ground turkey in a marinara sauce one night, toss the rest with some basic seasonings for a taco bowl another night. If you need only half a bunch of broccoli for broccoli cheddar soup, use the rest in a stir-fry or breakfast frittata.

Cross-utilizing ingredients saves you time by allowing you to prepare several meal's worth of a vegetable, grain or protein at one time (see page 39 for more timesaving tips). It also prevents waste. How many times have you used part of an onion or half a package of tortillas only to find the rest weeks later spoiled in your refrigerator or stale in your pantry? By overlapping the ingredients in your meals, you'll be able to use up what you buy.

Here are some suggestions for cross-utilizing ingredients. You'll find the recipes for many of these dishes in this cookbook.

Broccoli
- Egg bake or smoked Gouda frittata
- Broccoli cheddar soup
- Broccoli bites

	WEEK 1	WEEK 2	WEEK 3
VEGETABLES	Cauliflower	Broccoli	Cauliflower
	Zucchini	Zucchini	Green beans
	Carrots	Carrots	Carrots
	Bell peppers	Bell peppers	Bell peppers
GRAINS	Whole-grain pitas	Whole-grain tortillas	Whole-grain pitas
	Brown rice	Brown rice	Quinoa
	Whole-grain pasta	Whole-grain pasta	Whole-grain pasta
PROTEINS	Shrimp	Salmon	Salmon
	Lean ground beef	Lean ground beef	Pork tenderloin
	Chicken breast	Chicken breast	Chicken breast

- Stir-fry
- Penne pasta with marinara sauce or pesto

Bell peppers
- Fajitas
- Stir-fry
- Egg bake or omelet
- Vegetable kebabs
- Rice or quinoa pilaf

Green beans
- Green beans with almonds
- Minestrone soup
- Pasta salad

Cauliflower
- Garlic cauliflower mashed potatoes
- Parmesan-crusted cauliflower
- Egg frittata

Black beans
- Cuban black bean soup
- Three bean chili
- Veggie quesadillas
- Breakfast burritos
- Salads

- Beans and rice
- Black bean burgers

Chicken breasts
- Lemon chicken
- Chicken Parmesan
- Chicken salad sandwich
- Chicken wild rice soup
- Santa Fe lime chicken fajitas
- Stir-fry
- Tacos

Ground lean turkey, chicken or beef
- Swedish meatballs
- Shepherd's pie
- Southwest taco bowl
- Meatloaf
- Meaty pasta sauce
- Lasagna
- Burgers

Shrimp
- Coconut shrimp
- Tuscan shrimp
- Stir-fry
- Penne pasta with marinara sauce or pesto

MAKING THE MOST OF CHICKEN AND OTHER LEAN MEATS

Chicken breasts are a healthy, lean protein that work well in a variety of recipes. The problem is that many of the chicken breasts sold at grocery stores are much larger than a single serving. To cut a thick chicken breast down to size, butterfly it. This simply means slicing it lengthwise down the middle with your chef's knife. You'll end up with two thinner cuts of meat that will be better proportioned and take less time to cook.

If you're serving chicken or another lean meat as its own entree, with grains and veggies on the side, plan on cooking it the day you'll be eating it. It's juiciest and most flavorful right off the grill or out of the oven. Any lean meat you precook to use for later meals will taste best if cut up and mixed with other ingredients. Reheated meat tends to lose moisture and flavor, so it benefits from the juices and seasonings in dishes such as stir-fries and mixed salads.

Being efficient in the kitchen

Having a solid meal plan is an important step toward practical, healthy cooking. But, let's face it, all those ingredients aren't going to chop, mix and cook themselves. After a long day, many people don't look forward to the idea of making dinner. The thought of all that preparation and cooking can be exhausting. Fortunately, there's another way. Mealtime can be hassle-free if you implement a few simple kitchen strategies.

It starts with a shift in how you think about food preparation. The goal is to streamline the process at every turn. Each and every time you chop, mix, cook or bake, try to prepare extra to store and use later. Then, on busy days or hectic nights, all you need to do is grab and go. Some of your meals will be prepped ingredients that you're pulling from the fridge or freezer and combining. Others will be like your own frozen ready-to-eat meals that simply need to be heated.

The following strategies can save you time and energy and help turn your kitchen into a well-oiled machine.

Cross-utilize kitchen equipment

Cross-utilization isn't just for ingredients. You can also save time by multitasking with your kitchen equipment. If you're slicing up a batch of peppers for the week, take that opportunity to cut all your vegetables. Then you'll only have to clean your cutting board, knife and counters once.

Apply the same philosophy to cooking with your oven, grill or stovetop. When you're roasting a batch of chopped vegetables, why not also bake some sweet potatoes, Parmesan-crusted cauliflower or chicken for later in the week? If you're grilling some beef tenderloin for dinner, use the extra grill space to cook up some chicken or veggie kebabs for future meals. If you're using a pan to sauté onion and pepper slices for fajitas, sauté enough for a stir-fry later in the week.

By cross-utilizing your equipment, you'll consolidate your prep work and get the most time-consuming steps of the cooking process out of the way.

Plan your prep time

You're probably catching on to the idea that doing your food preparation in big batches is a big timesaver. Put that strategy into action by setting aside two times each week, including at least one weekend day, to do the majority of your prep work. At each prep session, work ahead on meals for the next few days. Starting on the next page are some suggestions for how to use your prep time efficiently.

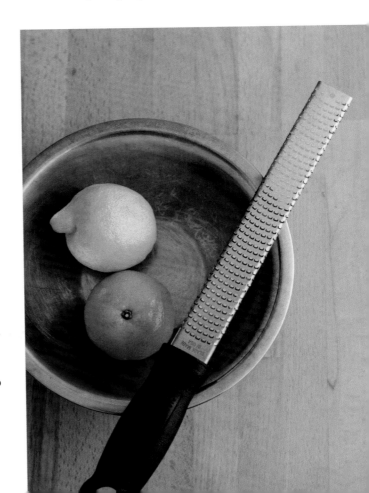

- PREP YOUR VEGGIES | Cut all your vegetables into shapes and sizes that will work for other meals in your weekly menu. That might mean slicing half your bell peppers for a stir-fry and dicing the other half for a rice pilaf. You can also get some cooking done ahead of time by roasting, sautéing or steaming vegetables to use in several of the week's recipes.
- MAKE YOUR GRAINS | Small grains such as pasta, rice and quinoa can be cooked ahead of time in larger batches to be divided up for several meals.
- COOK YOUR PROTEINS | Sear, grill and bake meats and plant-based proteins in batches to use over the next few days.

Store food wisely

Once you've cut your veggies and precooked some grains and a few nights' worth of meat, what do you do with all that food? The goal is to use it, not lose it somewhere in your refrigerator or freezer. Here's how.

PUT THE PEP IN PREP TIME

Your weekly prep sessions can be more enjoyable when you combine them with something entertaining. Stream a movie or TV show, listen to some upbeat music, or play an engaging podcast to help the time fly by.

Prep time can also be an opportunity for family time. Get the whole gang involved by assigning age-appropriate tasks. Maybe your spouse or partner helps you chop veggies while your children help you divide them up and pack them into containers. Not only will you be together, but you'll also be modeling lifelong kitchen habits.

Divvy it up

Rather than store a week's worth of cut vegetables in one container, divide the vegetables by meal. Store the onions and peppers for Monday's stir-fry separately from the peppers, carrots and zucchini for Tuesday's quinoa pilaf. The same goes for cooked grains. Portion them out for each separate meal. Store your ingredients in clear, stackable containers, sealable bags or a combination of the two.

This storage system means you'll have the right ingredients ready to go when mealtime rolls around. Portioning your ingredients ahead of time also makes it easier to manage the amount of each food group you're consuming.

Refrigerate

Set aside room in your refrigerator for the prepped ingredients you plan to use that week. How long can you store them safely? While many raw vegetables can last a week or more in the refrigerator, cooked vegetables, meats and grains should be eaten within three or four days. Just be sure to reheat any cooked meat until it reaches a safe internal temperature of 165 F.

Freeze

Freezing extra food is another way to save a lot of time in the long run — but not if you freeze it and forget it. (See the opposite page for freezing-ahead ideas.) Make a plan to use any food you're going to freeze. For example, if you freeze several weeks' worth of breaded chicken breasts, use them for one dinner each week over the next month.

A good rule of thumb is to use frozen foods within three months. Clearly date and label them, and keep a list of your freezer's contents. Periodically go through your freezer to remove foods that are unidentifiable or have been sitting in your freezer for too long.

Shortcuts in the kitchen

Looking for more ways to spend less time in the kitchen? Try some of these additional tips.

Make extra and freeze it

If you've got more cut vegetables than you can use in a week, consider blanching and freezing them to use later. This works best with harder veggies that have a lower water content, such as broccoli, cauliflower, green beans or carrots.

If you're making a more time-consuming dish for dinner, prepare extra to freeze and heat up later. This works well with many sauces and casseroles. Divide and freeze a sauce or dish in single servings or family-sized servings. Or bake casseroles in smaller aluminum tins that you can place directly in the freezer after cooling.

Freezing is also a good option for individual foods, such as breaded chicken breasts and uncooked pita pizzas. If you're assembling some for one meal, make four or five extra. Place them uncooked on a baking sheet or freezer-safe dish in the freezer. Once they're frozen, wrap them in plastic wrap to use later. On another night, unwrap what you need and bake it. For the best flavor and texture, place frozen items into the oven still frozen and bake at a high temperature of 425-450 F.

Make brown rice in batches

Brown rice is flavorful, healthy and filling, but it takes around 50 minutes to cook. To save time, make a large batch. When the rice is done, spread it out on a baking sheet to cool. Then put single or family-sized servings in sealable bags to store in the freezer.

If you're planning on mixing the frozen rice into a dish you're cooking, such as turkey wild rice soup or veggie rice pilaf, you can add the rice directly to the pot or pan. If you'll be

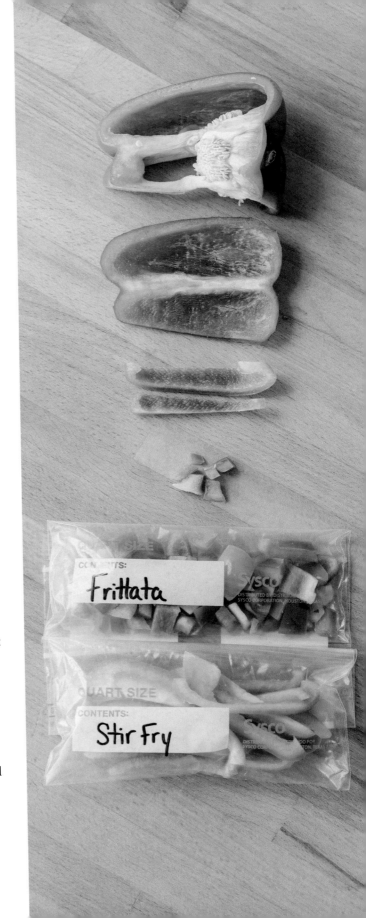

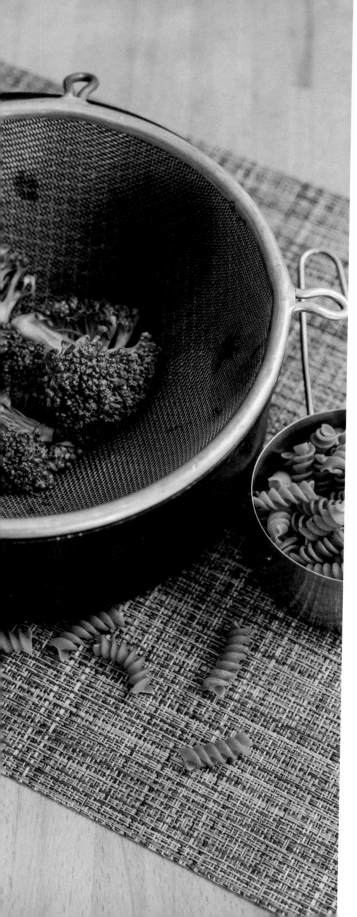

serving the rice on the side, microwave some water to boiling in a bowl or large measuring cup. Soak the rice in the hot water to heat it through, then drain. This not only warms up the rice but also rehydrates it and releases its natural flavors.

Pile on the pilaf
Pilaf is simply diced vegetables mixed with a small grain, such as brown rice, quinoa or whole-grain couscous. It's a versatile and filling dish that works well with a variety of ingredients and flavors. That makes it a great dish to prepare in big batches and use throughout the week.

If you're making pilaf for one meal, make enough for one or two more. Then separate it into halves or thirds and season each of those portions differently. For example, you could add thyme, cashews and dried cranberries to one portion and cumin and lime juice to another. The rest could go into chicken broth or canned soup. Don't be afraid to experiment. The sky's the limit.

Preserve your potatoes
If your menu plan includes potatoes a couple of nights during the week, you can cut them all at once and store them in containers of cold water in the refrigerator. When you need them, pat them dry, then season and cook them as you normally would.

Precook your pasta
If you're making pasta for dinner, make extra for later. You can store extra pasta in the refrigerator for a week or two. Have spaghetti with marina sauce one night. Another night toss the extra pasta with some vegetable oil, soy sauce and stir-fry vegetables to make lo mein.

Steam while you boil
If you're cooking pasta, rice or potatoes, you can multitask by steaming vegetables you

need at the same time you are preparing the pasta, rice or potatoes. Rest a wire mesh strainer on top of the pot and put cut vegetables in it. Place the pot's lid on top of the strainer and let the steam from the heated water do its job. You can also use this method when you're simmering soup. The flavor from the soup will add flavor to your veggies!

Purchase minimally processed, ready-to-go ingredients

If you're feeling short on time or less than confident about your skills with a chef's knife, consider buying some of your vegetables precut. Frozen vegetables are another option. Just make sure you're getting plain veggies and not ones drenched in sauce.

Another shortcut is parboiled brown rice. Parboiled rice takes about half as long to cook as regular brown rice. You can buy parboiled rice in stores or make your own. Cook brown rice halfway through and store it in the refrigerator and finish cooking it later in the week or freeze it for later use.

Use canned soup as a starter kit

Low-sodium, low-fat soup can be a great base for a healthy and hearty meal. Throw in your favorite ingredients, such as cooked brown rice or whole-grain pasta, diced vegetables, and precooked lean meat.

Use dinner ingredients for lunch

Don't view your leftovers in a bad light — they make a great lunch! As you're preparing your meals for the week, think about how you might use extra portions left over from the previous night's dinner.

If you want some variety, you can use your dinner ingredients in different ways. For example, take an unused tortilla from your dinner tacos to make a lunch wrap. Slice up an extra piece of grilled chicken breast for a sandwich or to use in Asian chicken salad.

Pace yourself

As you delve into the recipes in this cookbook, rely on the simple strategies outlined here and in the previous section to streamline your work. If the idea of preparing most of your weekly meals still seems overwhelming, know that you're not alone. It can take time and practice to get comfortable in the kitchen.

If you rarely cook for yourself, set realistic goals and begin with small steps. Start with two or three meals a week and gradually build from there. Another way to ease into cooking is to get to know a few recipes well before expanding your repertoire. Soon you'll become more confident in preparing your own foods and be more willing to explore a broader range of recipes.

If time is an issue for you, by utilizing a few kitchen shortcuts and some advance planning you can fit homemade meals into your busy schedule. Preparing healthy meals doesn't have to eat up all of your time. If you have children, you might establish a routine around mealtimes. Maybe a younger child assembles the dinner ingredients or sets the table while an older child helps chop the vegetables or prepare the pasta or rice.

Most of all, remember to have fun! There's no right or wrong in cooking. What matters is that you and your family become comfortable in the kitchen, and that you discover the good feelings and satisfaction that comes with creating flavorful and healthy meals for yourself and your family.

Finally, keep in mind that discovering new foods and flavors is part of the joy of cooking, so don't be afraid to explore unfamiliar recipes. Experiment, and let your taste buds lead the way. There's no better time to be adventurous!

Mixing and matching meals

Cross-utilization involves purchasing a set of ingredients to use in your meals throughout the week. Benefits are you purchase fewer items, reduce prep time and ensure food doesn't go to waste. Think about meals that call for the same vegetables, grains, and proteins and dairy and put them in the same weekly menu.

You can also practice cross-utilization without recipes. Just purchase some core ingredients and come up with different ways to combine them during the week, as shown in this sample chart. Ingredients are used in different and overlapping ways throughout the week.

INGREDIENTS FOR THE WEEK

Protein/dairy
- Chicken
- Cod
- Black beans
- Eggs
- Cheese (cheddar, feta, other)

Vegetables
- Peppers
- Onions
- Corn
- Tomatoes
- Zucchini
- Lettuce

Grains
- Brown rice
- Whole-wheat pasta
- Whole-wheat tortillas

	SUNDAY	MONDAY
BREAKFAST	**Omelet** Eggs Cheese Peppers Onions Tomatoes	**Breakfast burrito** Eggs Cheese Tomatoes Onions Peppers Whole-wheat tortillas
LUNCH	**Chicken wrap** Chicken breast Lettuce Tomato Pepper Whole-wheat tortillas	**Leftover chicken stir-fry**
DINNER	**Chicken stir-fry** Chicken breast Peppers Onions Brown rice	**Cuban black bean soup** Black beans Tomatoes Peppers Onions

TUESDAY	WEDNESDAY	THURSDAY	FRIDAY	SATURDAY
Omelet ▢ Eggs ▢ Cheese ● Peppers ● Onions ● Tomatoes	**Breakfast burrito** ▢ Eggs ▢ Cheese ● Tomatoes ● Onions ● Peppers ◆ Whole-wheat tortillas	**Egg scramble** ▢ Scrambled eggs with cheese ○ Zucchini ● Tomatoes	**Breakfast burrito** ▢ Eggs ▢ Cheese ● Tomatoes ● Onions ● Pepper ◆ Whole-wheat tortillas	**Egg scramble** ▢ Scrambled eggs with cheese ○ Zucchini ● Tomatoes
▍**Leftover Cuban black bean soup**	**Southwest taco chicken salad** ■ Black beans ■ Chicken ▢ Cheese ● Peppers ● Onions ● Tomatoes ● Lettuce	▍**Leftover chicken Parmesan and salad**	**Veggie panini wrap** ▢ Cheese ● Onions ○ Zucchini ● Peppers ● Lettuce ◆ Whole-wheat tortillas	**Fish quesadilla** ■ Cod ○ Corn ● Tomatoes ● Peppers ◆ Whole-wheat tortillas
Grilled fish with rice pilaf ■ Cod ○ Zucchini ● Peppers ● Onions ◆ Brown rice	▍**Chicken Parmesan with pasta and salad** ■ Chicken breast ● Lettuce ● Tomatoes ○ Zucchini ◆ Whole-wheat penne pasta	**Blackened fish tacos with black bean and corn salsa** ■ Cod ■ Black beans ○ Corn ● Tomatoes ◆ Whole-wheat tortillas	**Lemon chicken with penne pasta mixed with veggies** ■ Chicken breast ○ Zucchini ● Onions ◆ Whole-wheat penne pasta or ◆ Brown rice	**Chicken rice vegetable soup** ■ Chicken breast ◆ Brown rice Leftover vegetables

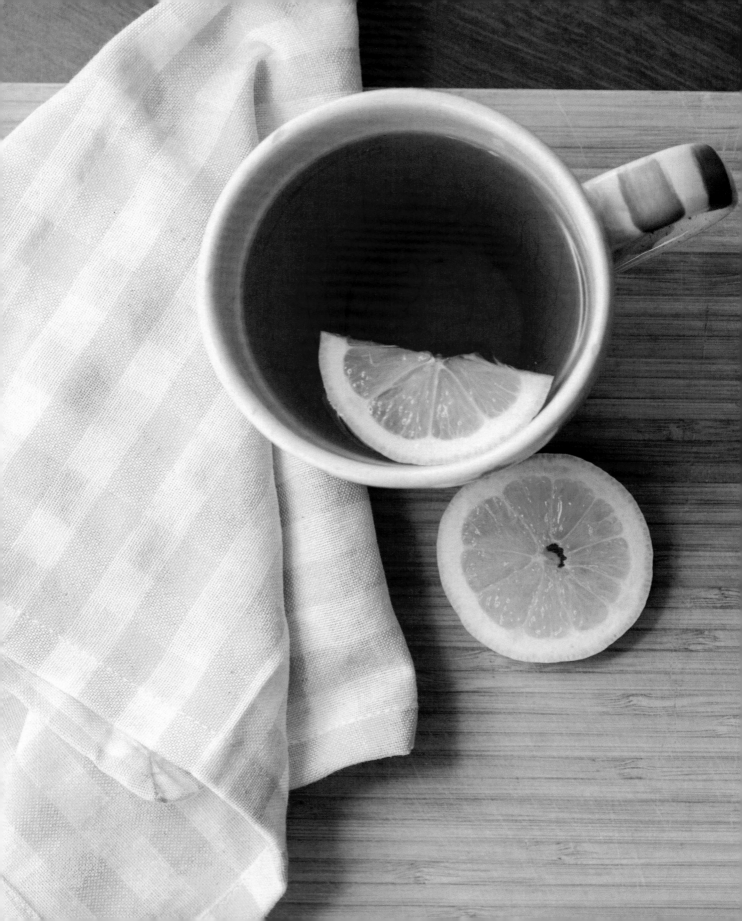

Breakfast

Banana flax pancakes

In addition to sliced bananas, enjoy these pancakes with fresh blueberries and a sprinkling of cinnamon or powdered sugar.

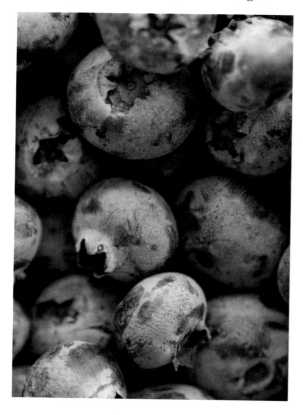

1 cup ground flaxseed
1 cup all-purpose flour
1 tablespoon baking powder
1 tablespoon sugar
½ teaspoon salt
1 ½ cups skim milk
2 eggs
1 teaspoon vanilla extract
1 ¼ cup mashed bananas

In a medium bowl, combine the flaxseed, flour, baking powder, sugar and salt. In another medium bowl, combine the milk, eggs and vanilla extract.

Make a small indentation (a "well") in the middle of the dry ingredients, and slowly add the wet ingredients to the dry while whisking. Add mashed bananas to the mixture.

Lightly coat a large sauté pan or griddle with cooking spray and preheat to medium heat. Place ¼-cup scoops of batter in the pan. The pancakes should be golden on each side.

Due to the heaviness of the flaxseed, these pancakes may take a longer time to cook through. Lower the heat, if necessary. A pancake is done when it feels firm to the touch instead of mushy.

SHOPPING LIST: Ground flaxseed, bananas

CHECK FOR: All-purpose flour, baking powder, sugar, salt, skim milk, eggs, vanilla, cooking spray

NUTRITIONAL ANALYSIS PER SERVING
(1 PANCAKE): 130 calories, 4 g fat, 5 g protein, 18 g carbohydrates, 3 g fiber, 170 mg sodium

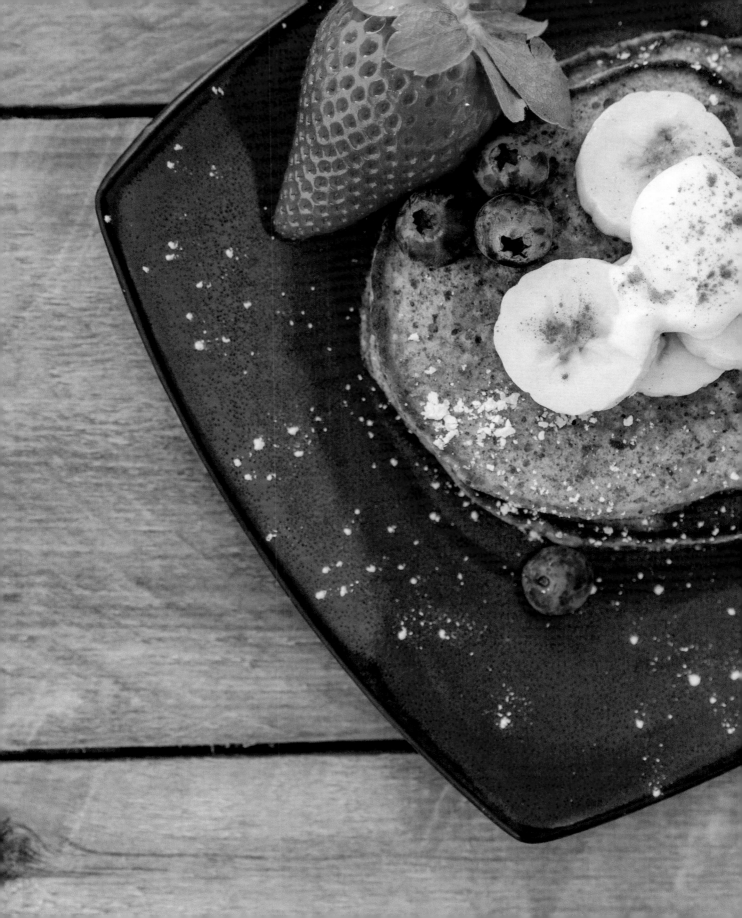

Cinnamon carrot pancakes

Substituting 2 cups of pumpkin purée for the carrots in this recipe makes for a wonderful fall breakfast.

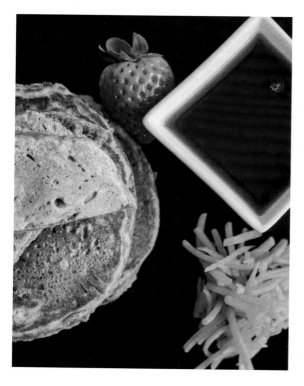

1 ½ cups all-purpose flour
½ cup ground flaxseed
1 ¾ cup skim milk
2 large eggs
2 tablespoons canola oil
2 tablespoons baking powder
1 teaspoon salt
1 teaspoon vanilla extract
5 tablespoons sugar
¼ teaspoon nutmeg
2 teaspoons cinnamon
¼ teaspoon ground cloves
3 cups shredded carrots

In a medium bowl, combine dry ingredients: flour, flaxseed, baking powder, salt, sugar and spices. Mix well.

In a separate bowl, combine skim milk, eggs and canola oil. Mix well.

Create a small well in the dry mixture. Slowly add the wet mix to the dry mix, carefully whisking together while combining. Add in the shredded carrots.

Lightly spray a sauté pan or griddle with cooking spray and preheat to medium heat. Use a ¼-cup scoop to measure out each pancake. Place in the pan or on the griddle and slowly cook until done all the way through. The pancakes should be golden on each side. These pancakes are thicker and will need time on each side to cook through. Lower the heat if necessary. The pancakes should feel firm to the touch and not mushy.

SHOPPING LIST: Ground flaxseed, carrots

CHECK FOR: All-purpose flour, skim milk, eggs, canola oil, baking powder, salt, vanilla, sugar, nutmeg, cinnamon, ground cloves, cooking spray

NUTRITIONAL ANALYSIS PER SERVING
(1 PANCAKE): 100 calories, 2 g fat, 4 g protein, 18 g carbohydrates, 2 g fiber, 360 mg sodium

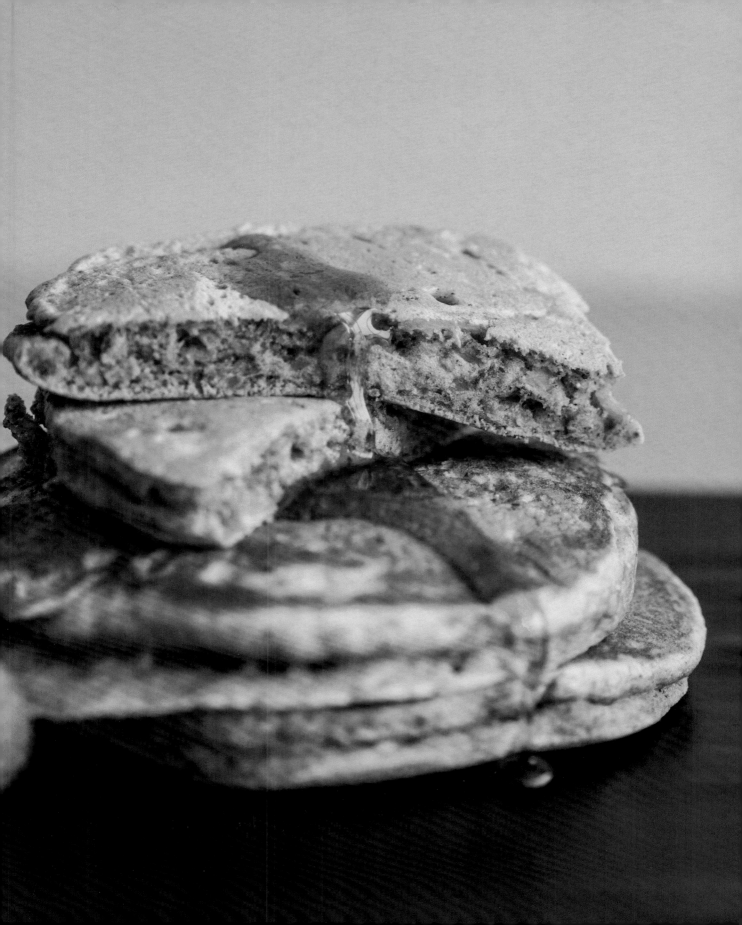

Blueberry pancakes

SERVINGS: 8 |

All-purpose flour is used to help keep the pancakes light. Wheat germ adds fiber and creates the full feeling you get when eating these pancakes. Different fruits may be substituted for blueberries in this recipe.

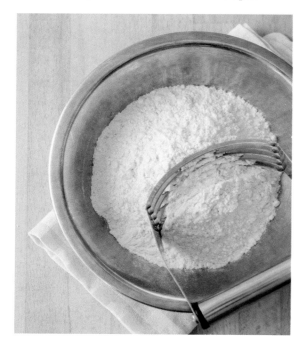

SHOPPING LIST: Wheat germ or ground flaxseed, Greek yogurt, blueberries

CHECK FOR: All-purpose flour, sugar, baking powder, salt, eggs, skim milk, vanilla, cooking spray

NUTRITIONAL ANALYSIS PER SERVING
(1 PANCAKE): 160 calories, 4 g fat, 7 g protein, 23 g carbohydrates, 2 g fiber, 220 mg sodium

1 cup all-purpose flour
¾ cup wheat germ or ground flaxseed
2 tablespoons sugar
1 teaspoon baking powder
½ teaspoon salt
2 large eggs
½ cup skim milk
½ cup fat-free plain Greek yogurt
2 teaspoons vanilla extract
1 cup fresh or frozen blueberries

In medium bowl, mix all dry ingredients. In separate bowl, combine all wet ingredients.

Create a small well in the middle of the dry ingredients and slowly whisk together the wet ingredients with the dry.

Place fresh or frozen blueberries into the batter and mix lightly.

Lightly spray a sauté pan or griddle with cooking spray and preheat to medium heat. Place ¼-cup scoops of batter in the pan. Pancakes will be about 4 inches in circumference.

Cook until lightly golden on each side. Should take about 2-3 minutes on each side. It's important not to rush the process of cooking. Higher heat will not help cook the pancakes all the way through.

Roasted sweet potato hash

SERVINGS: 4 |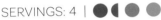

Butternut squash can be added to or substituted for sweet potatoes in this hash. Other vegetables also work well in a hash! You can use what you have on hand — all that matters is that it's nutrient dense and tastes great. Try adding kale, mushrooms, poblano peppers, green onions, baby red potatoes and celery.

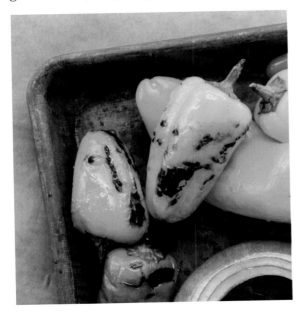

SHOPPING LIST: Sweet potatoes, onion, red bell pepper, green bell pepper, jalapeno pepper, chicken sausage, fresh rosemary, fresh thyme

CHECK FOR: Olive oil, kosher salt, pepper, cooking spray

NUTRITIONAL ANALYSIS PER SERVING (1 CUP): 210 calories, 6 g fat, 1 g saturated fat, 14 g protein, 28 g carbohydrate, 5 g fiber, 220 mg sodium

2 cups peeled and cubed sweet potatoes, cut into 1- to 2-inch chunks
1 medium onion of any color, chopped
1 red bell pepper, chopped
1 green bell pepper, chopped
1 jalapeno, minced (optional)
8 ounces chicken sausage
1 tablespoon chopped fresh rosemary
1 tablespoon chopped fresh thyme
1 tablespoon olive oil
½ teaspoon kosher salt
¼ teaspoon ground black pepper

Preheat oven to 400 F. Lightly spray a baking pan with cooking spray or coat with oil. Cube the sweet potatoes and set aside.

Chop the onion, bell peppers, jalapeno pepper and fresh herbs and place in a medium-sized bowl. Add the oil, salt and pepper. Add the sweet potatoes and chicken sausage and mix well.

Place the mixture on the prepared pan. Roast in the oven for approximately 20 minutes. At 10 minutes, flip the sweet potatoes and sausage to aid in even browning.

Breakfast potatoes

SERVINGS: 6 |

Sprinkle the potatoes with paprika before roasting them in the oven to add more color. These breakfast potatoes are a great side with any lean source of protein.

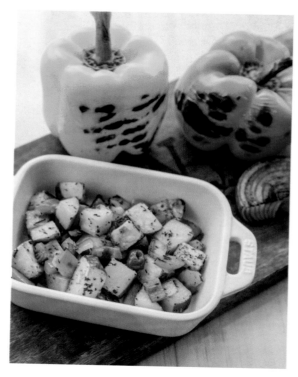

SHOPPING LIST: Russet potatoes, onions, green bell pepper, red bell pepper

CHECK FOR: Onion powder, garlic powder, salt, pepper, olive oil, cooking spray

NUTRITIONAL ANALYSIS PER SERVING
(½ CUP): 190 calories, 2 g fat, 5 g protein, 39 g carbohydrates, 5 g fiber, 200 mg sodium

3 large russet potatoes
1 ½ medium onions, finely chopped
⅓ cup chopped green pepper
⅓ cup chopped red pepper
1 tablespoon olive oil
1 teaspoon onion powder
1 teaspoon garlic powder
1 teaspoon salt
½ teaspoon ground black pepper
½ teaspoon olive oil

Preheat oven to 400 F. Lightly coat a baking sheet with cooking spray. Cut each potato into 1-inch chunks.

In a medium bowl, combine 1 tablespoon oil, onion powder, garlic powder, salt and pepper. Place the potatoes in the bowl and evenly coat them with the seasoning mix. Place the potatoes on the prepared baking sheet. Roast in the oven for 20-30 minutes. Every 10 minutes, use a spatula to turn the potatoes to evenly brown them.

Add ½ teaspoon oil to a sauté pan and heat to medium high. Sauté the onions and peppers for approximately 5-7 minutes or until tender. Set the pan aside and cover to keep warm.

When the potatoes are done, toss with the onions and peppers and serve.

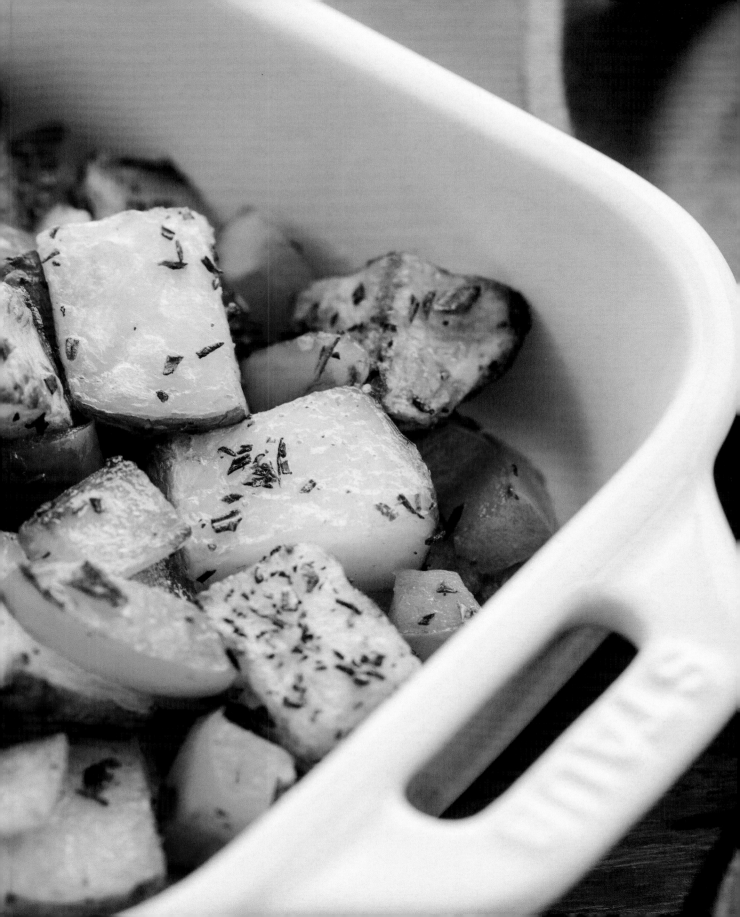

Cheesy poached egg sandwich

SERVINGS: 6 | ● ●

For a variation, on an English muffin place a slice of fresh mozzarella cheese and a serving of the tomato mixture used in tomato bruschetta (see page 103) and top with a poached egg.

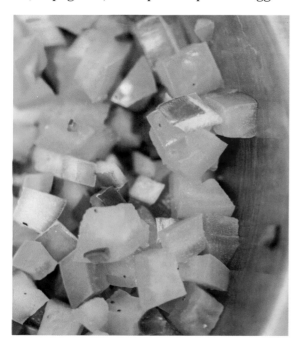

SHOPPING LIST: Roma tomatoes, cilantro, lime, shredded sharp cheddar cheese, onion, jalapeno pepper, whole-wheat English muffins

CHECK FOR: Salt , white vinegar, eggs, kosher salt, pepper

NUTRITIONAL ANALYSIS PER SERVING (1 SANDWICH): 210 calories, 10 g fat, 4.5 g saturated fat, 13 g protein, 18 g carbohydrates, 1 g fiber, 360 mg sodium

1 cup chopped Roma tomatoes
¼ cup minced onion
1 tablespoon chopped fresh cilantro
1 jalapeno pepper, minced
1 lime, juiced
Pinch of salt
3 whole-wheat English muffins
3 ounces shredded sharp cheddar cheese
6 cups water
6 large eggs
1 tablespoon white vinegar
¼ teaspoon kosher salt
Ground black pepper

Preheat oven to 425 F, or you can use a toaster oven.

In a medium bowl, combine tomatoes, onions, cilantro, jalapeno pepper and lime juice. Add a pinch of salt to taste; set aside. Cut the English muffins in half and top with cheese. Place on a baking sheet and bake in a toaster oven or in a regular oven for about 5 minutes.

To prepare the eggs, in a medium-shallow pan, bring water to a boil. Add the vinegar. Slowly crack the eggs and add to the pan one at a time; cook to desired doneness. Eggs that have runny yolks take about 3-4 minutes.

Using a slotted spoon, retrieve the eggs from the water. Place tomato mixture (pico de gallo) on each muffin half and top with egg. Sprinkle with kosher salt and ground black pepper.

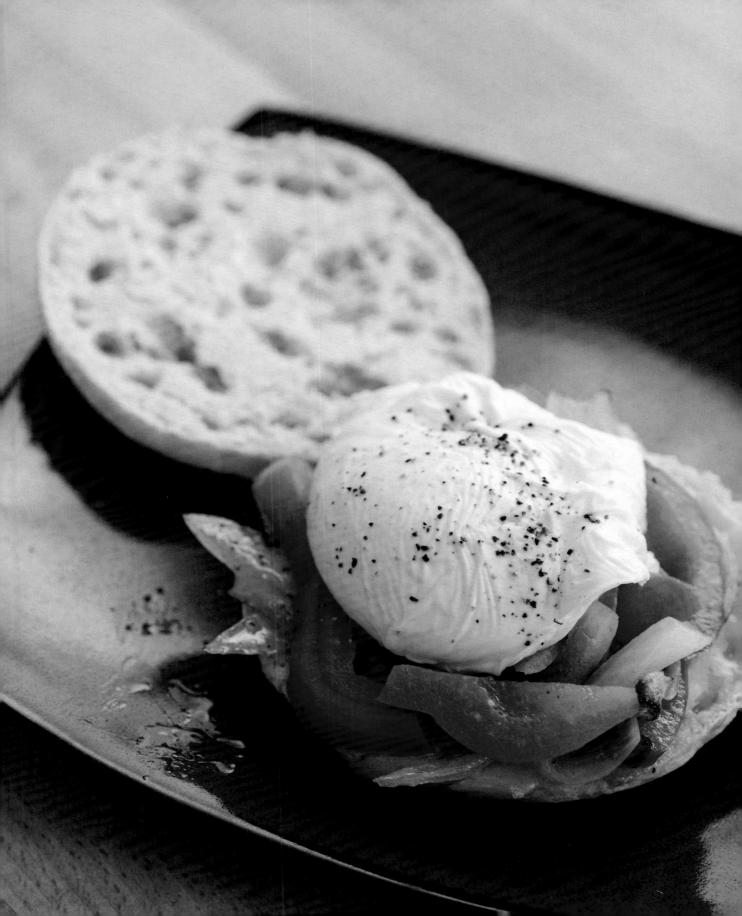

Chicken or turkey sausage patties

SERVINGS: 5 |

With chicken or turkey breast, you don't want to overcook the patties, which will dry them out. Using a thermometer is key. Make sure not to cook the patties over 165 F. When this recipe becomes a family favorite, you can double or triple the recipe and freeze the extra patties. Pull out what you need and quickly reheat them.

SHOPPING LIST: Garlic, onion, ground fennel, ground or fresh sage, maple syrup, ground chicken or turkey breast

CHECK FOR: Kosher salt, pepper, eggs, cooking spray

NUTRITIONAL ANALYSIS PER SERVING
(1 PATTY): 140 calories, 3.5 g fat, 1 g saturated fat, 21 g protein, 4 g carbohydrates, 240 mg sodium

2 teaspoons minced garlic
½ cup minced onion
¾ teaspoon ground fennel
1 teaspoon ground sage or 1 tablespoon finely
    chopped fresh sage
1 tablespoon maple syrup or brown sugar
½ teaspoon kosher salt
¼ teaspoon ground black pepper
1 pound ground chicken (or turkey) breast
1 large egg yolk

Preheat oven to 350 F. Preheat a medium- to large-sized nonstick pan to medium heat. When warm, sauté the onions and garlic, cooking 3-4 minutes until tender.

Remove from heat and place the onions and garlic in a medium bowl. Add fennel, sage, maple syrup or brown sugar, salt, pepper and egg yolk and mix well. Add chicken to mixture and gently combine ingredients with hands. Form into five 1-inch thick patties.

Lightly spray a nonstick pan with cooking spray or brush with oil. Preheat to medium heat.

Place each patty in preheated pan to create a nice sear. Sear about 1-2 minutes on each side, then place on a baking sheet. Bake approximately 10 minutes to an internal temperature of 165 F. You can also finish cooking the sausage in the pan but will need to reduce the heat to prevent burning due to the limited fat content.

Power morning muffins

SERVINGS: 24 | ◖◖

Use fat-free plain Greek yogurt to boost the protein in this recipe. Another way to prepare these muffins is to substitute shredded carrots for the blueberries.

SHOPPING LIST: Whole-wheat flour, ground flaxseed, unsalted butter, plain fat-free yogurt, fresh blueberries

CHECK FOR: All-purpose flour, baking powder, baking soda, salt, sugar, vanilla, eggs, cooking spray

NUTRITIONAL ANALYSIS PER SERVING (1 MUFFIN): 120 calories, 4.5 g fat, 2 g saturated fat, 3 g protein, 19 g carbohydrates, 2 g fiber, 40 mg sodium

1 ½ cups all-purpose flour
1 cup whole-wheat flour
½ cup ground flaxseed
1 tablespoon baking powder
½ teaspoon baking soda
½ tablespoon salt
3 ounces unsalted butter
1 cup sugar
½ tablespoon vanilla extract
2 eggs
1 cup plain fat-free yogurt
2 cups fresh blueberries

Preheat oven to 350 F. Combine both flours, flaxseed, baking powder, baking soda and salt in a bowl; set aside.

Using a stand or hand-held mixer, combine unsalted butter and sugar until creamy. Add the vanilla extract. Add one egg at a time. Then add the dry mixture, alternating it with the yogurt. Mix until well combined. Gently fold the blueberries into the mixture.

Lightly spray a muffin tin with cooking spray. Use a ¼-cup scoop to fill muffin cups. Bake 15-20 minutes until tops are golden or a toothpick inserted into a muffin comes out clean.

Orange cinnamon French toast

A variation of this recipe uses apple juice in place of the orange juice, along with 1 cup of diced apples. Pair this with a serving of caprese frittata for a complete breakfast.

SHOPPING LIST: Whole-wheat bread, orange juice

CHECK FOR: Eggs, vanilla, cinnamon, skim milk, brown sugar, cooking spray

NUTRITIONAL ANALYSIS PER SERVING
(1 PIECE): 220 calories, 6 g fat, 1.5 g saturated fat, 13 g protein, 29 g carbohydrates, 240 mg sodium

8 slices whole-wheat bread
8 eggs
8 ounces orange juice
2 teaspoons vanilla extract
1 teaspoon ground cinnamon
8 ounces skim milk
2 tablespoons brown sugar

Prepare a loaf pan by lightly spraying with cooking spray. Break up whole-wheat bread into chunks and place in prepared loaf pan.

In a medium mixing bowl, combine eggs, orange juice, vanilla, cinnamon, skim milk and brown sugar and whisk until well combined. Pour egg mixture over the whole-wheat bread.

Wrap with plastic wrap and then foil and let sit in refrigerator overnight.

The following morning, preheat oven to 350 F. Place in oven still covered for 30 minutes, then bake uncovered for an additional 10-15 minutes until lightly browned on top.

When done baking, place the pan onto its side and let French toast fall out. Cut while still hot and serve immediately.

Whole-wheat French toast

SERVINGS: 6 |

This is a traditional French toast recipe that can easily be dressed up with a fresh fruit compote (see pages 244 and 246). Use your bruised and imperfect fruit to make a compote.

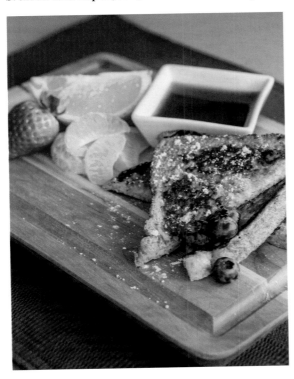

1 cup skim milk
½ cup egg substitute
1 egg
1 teaspoon vanilla extract
1 teaspoon ground cinnamon
⅛ teaspoon ground cloves
6 slices whole-wheat bread

Lightly coat a large sauté pan or griddle with cooking spray and preheat to medium-high heat.

In a medium mixing bowl, combine the milk, egg substitute, egg, vanilla, cinnamon and cloves.

Dip each slice of bread into the egg mixture until covered. Then place the bread in the sauté pan or on a griddle and cook approximately 1 ½ minutes or until golden brown. Using a spatula, flip the bread over and cook another 1 ½ minutes.

Serve with fresh fruit compote, fresh fruit, a sprinkle of powdered sugar or maple syrup.

SHOPPING LIST: Egg substitute, whole-wheat bread

CHECK FOR: Skim milk, eggs, vanilla, cinnamon, cloves, cooking spray

NUTRITIONAL ANALYSIS PER SERVING
(1 PIECE): 150 calories, 4 g fat, 1 g saturated fat, 10 g protein, 21 g carbohydrates, 200 mg sodium

Broccoli and smoked Gouda frittata

SERVINGS: 6 | ◖●●●

For variation, you can substitute cauliflower or asparagus for the broccoli and pepper jack or extra sharp cheddar cheese for one or both of the cheeses. Plain yogurt and raspberries make a good accompaniment.

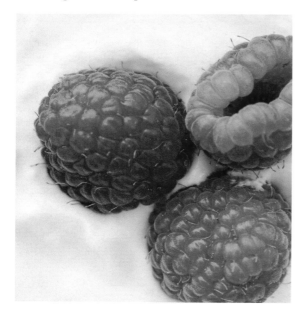

SHOPPING LIST: Broccoli, plain fat-free Greek yogurt, Dijon mustard, chives, sharp cheddar cheese, smoked Gouda cheese

CHECK FOR: Eggs, paprika, salt, pepper, olive oil

NUTRITIONAL ANALYSIS PER SERVING (1 WEDGE): 190 calories, 12 g fat, 6 g saturated fat, 17 g protein, 4 g carbohydrates, 1 g fiber, 640 mg sodium

1 small broccoli, cut into medium-small florets
6 eggs
¼ cup plain fat-free Greek yogurt
2 tablespoons Dijon mustard
2 teaspoons sweet paprika
3 tablespoons finely chopped chives
¼ cup shredded sharp cheddar cheese
½ cup smoked Gouda cheese
¼ teaspoon salt
¼ teaspoon ground black pepper
1 teaspoon olive oil

Simmer broccoli in a large pan of boiling salted water for 4-5 minutes, or until partially cooked. Drain and dry.

Preheat oven to 375 F. Break eggs into large bowl. Add the yogurt, mustard and paprika and whisk until thoroughly blended. Stir in the chives and half of the cheeses, and season with salt and pepper.

Heat the olive oil in large ovenproof frying pan. Fry the broccoli for about 5 minutes (until browned on one side). Pour the egg mixture over the broccoli. Use a fork to spread the broccoli evenly throughout the pan. Cook at medium heat for about 5 minutes. Scatter the remaining cheese on top.

Carefully transfer the pan to the oven. Cook 10-12 minutes or until the frittata is set. Remove from oven and rest 2-3 minutes before slicing into 6 wedges.

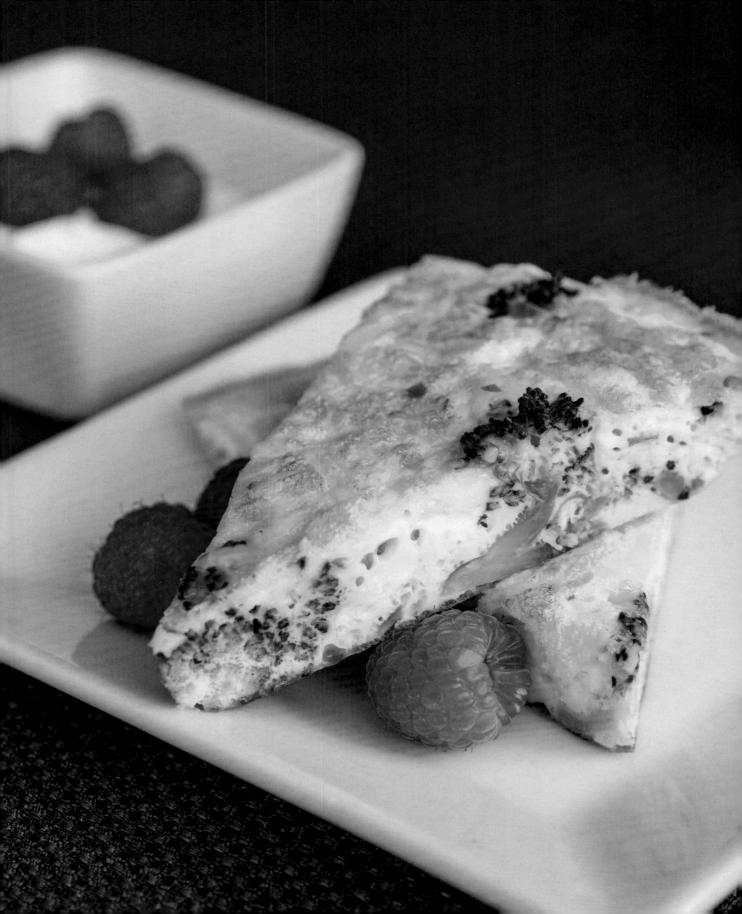

Caprese frittata

SERVINGS: 6 |

You can use any type of tomato, but ripe globe or beefsteak tomatoes are great choices. If you don't have fresh basil, substitute 1 tablespoon dried basil, although the flavor will be different. If you want a cheesier presentation, instead of including the cheese in the egg mixture, place it on top of the frittata before baking.

SHOPPING LIST: Globe tomatoes, egg whites, fresh basil, garlic, feta cheese crumbles, mozzarella cheese

CHECK FOR: Eggs, kosher salt, pepper, cooking spray

NUTRITIONAL ANALYSIS PER SERVING
(1 PIECE): 200 calories, 10 g fat, 5 g saturated fat, 22 g protein, 4 g carbohydrates, 580 mg sodium

2 globe tomatoes, washed and sliced
2 cups egg whites
6 eggs
4 tablespoons chopped fresh basil
1 tablespoon minced fresh garlic
½ cup feta cheese crumbles
1 cup shredded mozzarella cheese
½ teaspoon kosher salt
¼ teaspoon ground black pepper

Preheat oven to 375 F. Lightly spray an ovenproof skillet or baking pan with cooking spray. Prepare the tomatoes and set aside.

Place the eggs and egg whites in a mixing bowl and whisk them together. Gradually add the basil, garlic, cheeses, salt and pepper.

In the prepared skillet or baking pan, combine the egg mixture and sliced tomatoes. Cover with parchment paper and foil and bake for about 20 minutes.

Check the frittata. If the egg mixture is fairly set, then remove the foil and place the frittata back in the oven uncovered for about 5 minutes. When ready, cut into 6 wedges or squares and serve.

Frittatas hold up well in the refrigerator for several days. You can reheat leftovers for breakfast or lunch during the week.

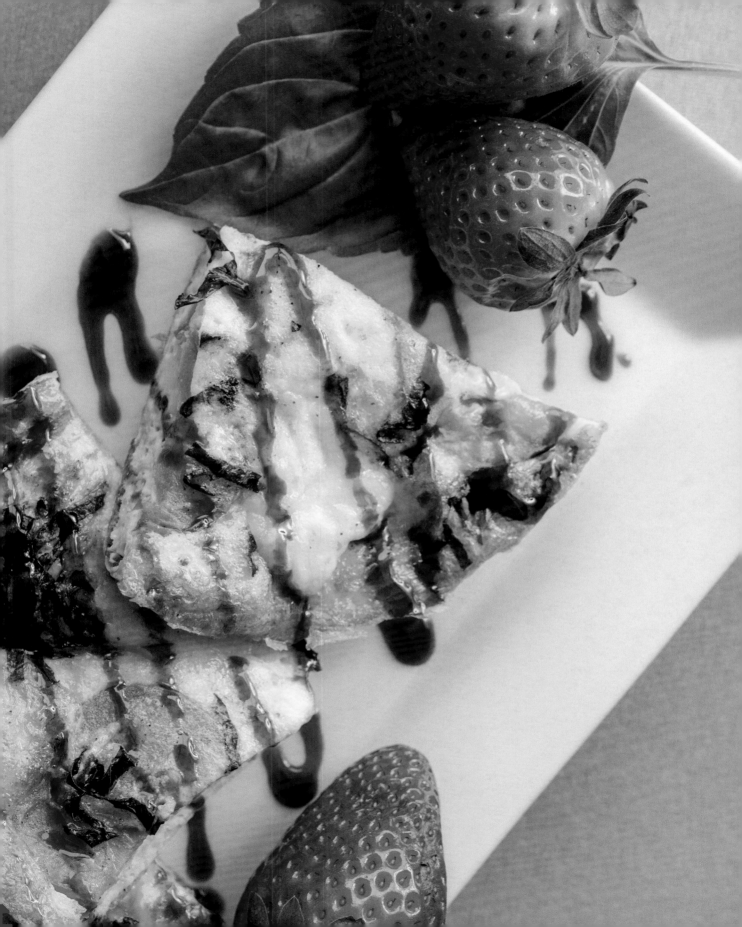

Southwest frittata

SERVINGS: 6 |

You can use leftover meat from the southwest taco bowl recipe (see page 182) in this frittata. Other vegetables that would work well in this frittata include onions, zucchini, tomatoes, mushrooms or eggplant. For different tastes, divide your pan into two different styles of frittata by moving or placing certain vegetables to one side or the other and changing up the cheeses.

SHOPPING LIST: Ground chicken breast, red bell pepper, green bell pepper, poblano pepper, pepper jack cheese

CHECK FOR: Paprika, cumin, garlic powder, onion powder, kosher salt, chili powder, oregano, cayenne pepper, eggs, skim milk, olive oil

NUTRITIONAL ANALYSIS PER SERVING (1 PIECE): 220 calories, 11 g fat, 5 g saturated fat, 21 g protein, 8 g carbohydrates, 2 g fiber, 540 mg sodium

8 ounces ground chicken breast
1 teaspoon olive oil
2 teaspoons paprika
2 teaspoons ground cumin
1 teaspoon garlic powder
1 teaspoon onion powder
1 teaspoon kosher salt
¼ teaspoon chili powder
½ teaspoon dried oregano
¼ teaspoon cayenne pepper
1 red bell pepper, chopped
1 green bell pepper, chopped
3 poblano peppers, chopped
2 tablespoons water
8 eggs
1 cup skim milk
3 ounces pepper jack cheese, shredded

Preheat oven to 375 F.

Heat a medium-sized ovenproof pan to medium-high heat. Sauté ground chicken breast in the olive oil. When chicken is browned, add the chopped peppers and sauté about 2-3 minutes. Add the spices, stirring frequently. Add about 2 tablespoons of water to help hydrate the spices.

Break eggs into large bowl and add the skim milk. Whisk until evenly blended. Pour eggs over sautéed ground chicken breast. Spread shredded pepper jack on top.

Carefully transfer the pan to the oven. Cook 10-12 minutes or until the frittata is set. Remove from oven and rest 2-3 minutes. Slice into 6 wedges or squares.

Cranberry apple oatmeal

SERVINGS: 6 |

Pick a sweeter apple for this dish to help balance the tartness of the cranberries. In place of the apple, you can use peaches, pears, plums, nectarines or blueberries. Make extra oatmeal for busy mornings during the week. For variety, make a batch without the fruit and use different fruit daily. If you'd prefer, you can leave out the brown sugar or substitute it with a local honey.

2 cups water
2 cups skim milk
1 cup oats
½ cup wheat bran
1 apple, diced (leave skin on)
1 cup frozen or fresh cranberries
2 tablespoons brown sugar
1 teaspoon ground cinnamon
1 teaspoon vanilla extract
¼ teaspoon ground cloves

In medium pot, bring water and milk to a boil. Add oats and wheat bran and cook about 3-5 minutes.

Stir in diced apple, cranberries, brown sugar, cinnamon, vanilla and cloves.

Cook for an additional 3 minutes or until oatmeal reaches desired consistency.

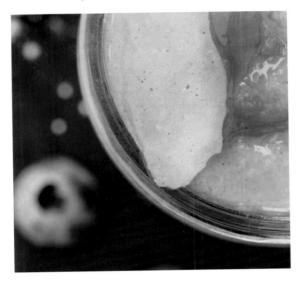

SHOPPING LIST: Oats, wheat bran, apple, cranberries

CHECK FOR: Skim milk, brown sugar, cinnamon, vanilla, cloves

NUTRITIONAL ANALYSIS PER SERVING (APPROX. 1 CUP): 140 calories, 1.5 g fat, 5 g protein, 28 g carbohydrates, 5 g fiber, 50 mg sodium

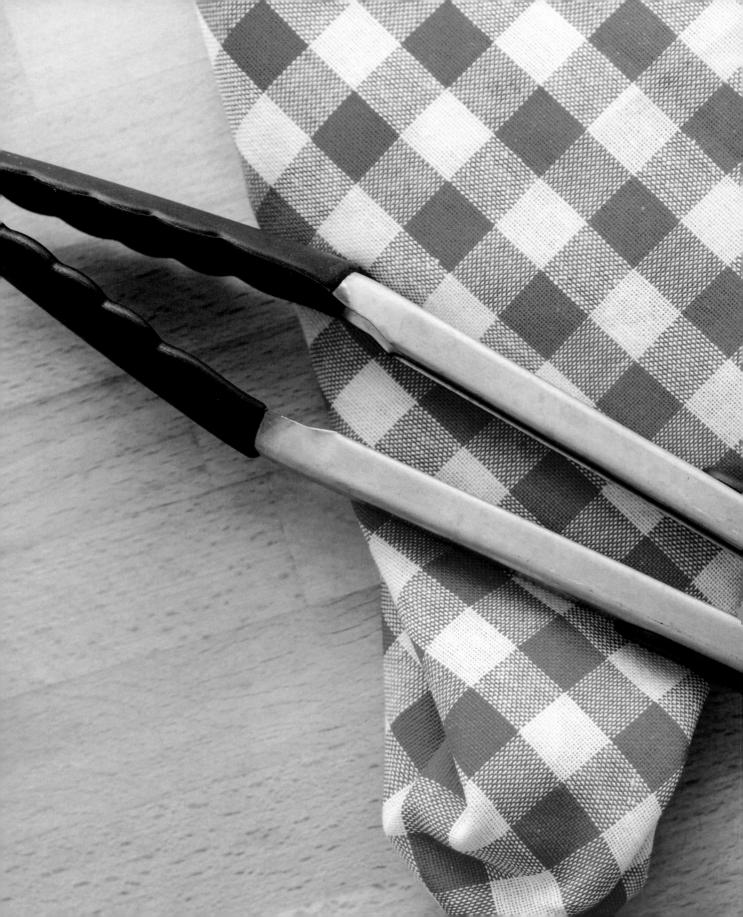

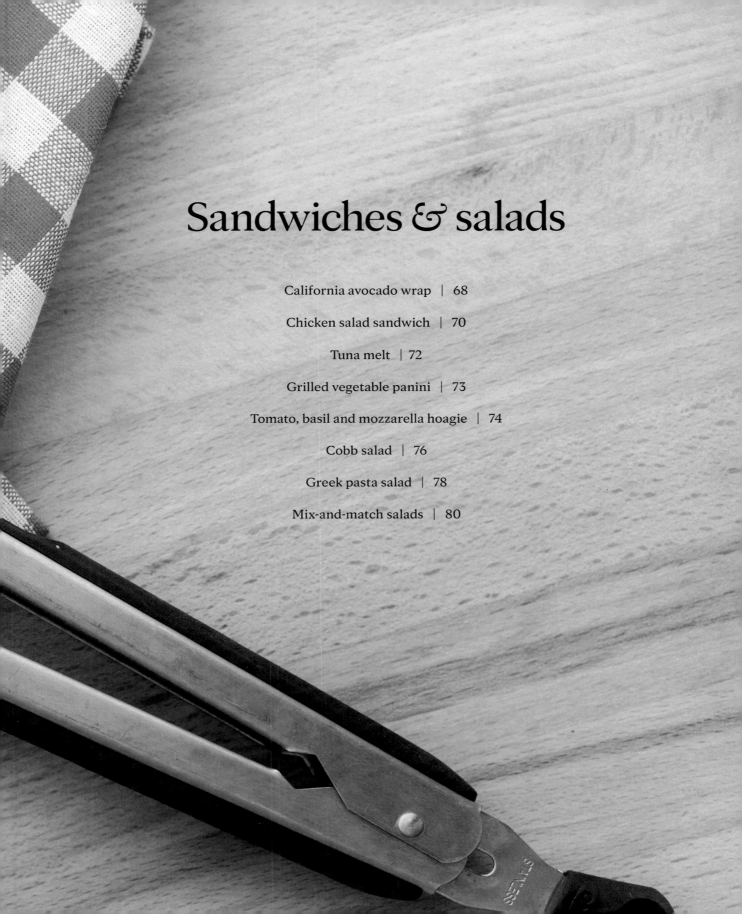

Sandwiches & salads

California avocado wrap

SERVINGS: 2 | ● ● ● ● ●●

A delicious variation to this recipe is to add a thin slice of 2% colby jack cheese to each wrap.

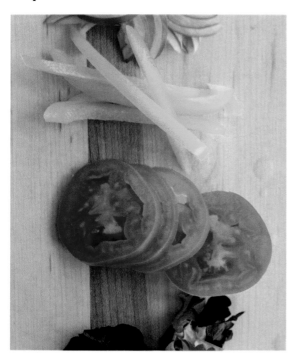

SHOPPING LIST: Whole-wheat tortillas, avocado, lime juice, Roma tomato, romaine lettuce, red onion, yellow bell pepper, chicken breast, ranch dressing

CHECK FOR: Salt

NUTRITIONAL ANALYSIS PER SERVING (1 WRAP): 410 calories, 14 g fat, 2.5 g saturated fat, 35 g protein, 38 g carbohydrates, 6 g fiber, 510 mg sodium

1 (14-inch) whole-wheat tortilla
½ avocado, sliced or mashed with lime juice and a pinch of salt
1 Roma tomato
2 leaves romaine lettuce
½ red onion, julienned
½ yellow bell pepper, julienned
6 ounces boneless, skinless chicken breast
1 ounce ranch dressing

Preheat a grill. Place the chicken on a hot grill. Cook 4-5 minutes on one side, then turn and cook an additional 4-5 minutes on the other side. Turn the chicken over to the first side so the grill makes a crisscross pattern and repeat on other side. (Cooking each side in two directions like this will give you great grill marks.) Once the chicken is thoroughly cooked, reaching an internal temperature of 165 F, remove it from the grill and cut into 6 strips. Set aside.

Cut the tortilla in half. Steam the tortilla halves by placing them on a plate and covering them with plastic wrap. Microwave for a few seconds.

Remove the tortilla halves from the microwave and put each on a plate. Spread each with ranch dressing and top with the rest of the ingredients.

Wrap up each tortilla half and stick it with a toothpick to hold it together.

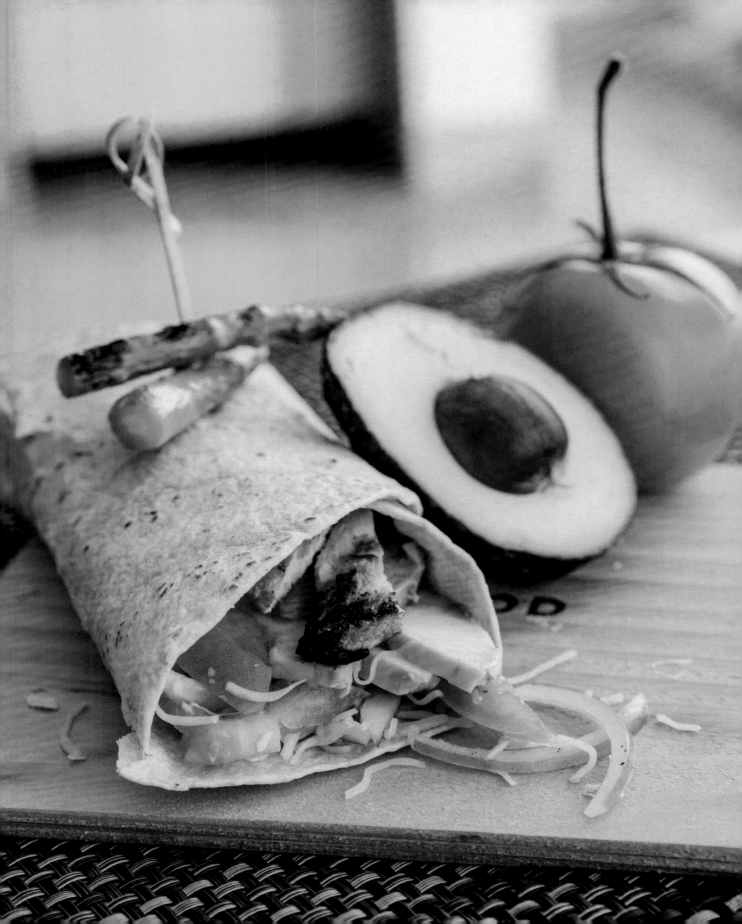

Chicken salad sandwich

If you're using whole chicken breasts larger than 4 ounces, butterfly them open so they're the proper size. Grill the chicken ahead of time for fast assembly. This is a great opportunity to make extra chicken and turkey bacon and refrigerate or freeze them for later use.

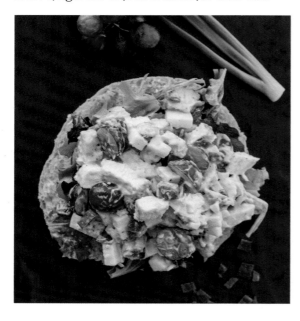

SHOPPING LIST: Chicken breasts, mayonnaise, celery, green onions, turkey bacon, red grapes, Swiss or Gruyére cheese, whole-wheat bread or sandwich thins, lettuce, tomato, red onion

CHECK FOR: Sea salt, white pepper, onion powder

NUTRITIONAL ANALYSIS PER SERVING (1 SANDWICH): 310 calories, 11 g fat, 3.5 g saturated fat, 29 g protein, 24 g carbohydrates, 460 mg sodium

2 small boneless, skinless chicken breasts, 4 ounces each
¼ teaspoon sea salt
¼ teaspoon white pepper
¼ teaspoon onion powder
¼ cup low-fat mayonnaise
¼ cup finely diced celery
1 tablespoon finely chopped green onions (finely chop the bottom bulbs)
4 pieces turkey bacon, cooked crisp and chopped
4 ounces red grapes, washed and sliced
2 ounces Swiss or Gruyére cheese, shredded or cubed
4 slices whole-wheat bread or sandwich thins
4 leaves lettuce
4 slices tomato
4 thin slices red onion

Preheat a grill. Season the chicken breasts with salt, pepper and onion powder. Grill the chicken over medium heat. A 3- to 4-ounce chicken breast should take approximately 4-5 minutes on each side to reach an internal temperature of 165 F. Remove from heat and chop the chicken into ½-inch to 1-inch sized pieces. (If you're making extra chicken, set it aside before chopping.)

If you haven't already done so, cook the turkey bacon until crispy. Mix together the chicken, mayo, celery, green onions, turkey bacon, grapes, cheese, and some salt and pepper.

Place the chicken salad mixture on 2 pieces of bread and spread out. Top each with lettuce, tomato, onion and another piece of bread. Cut each sandwich in half diagonally and serve.

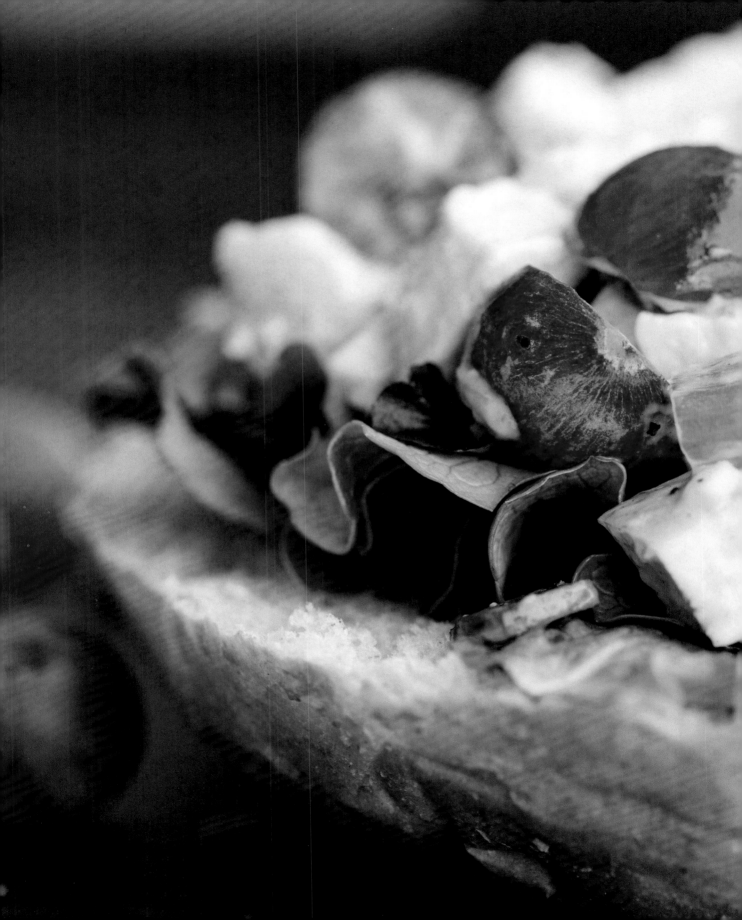

Tuna melt

SERVINGS: 4 | ◖ ● ●

When purchasing reduced-fat mayonnaise, look for brands that contain fewer ingredients.

SHOPPING LIST: Canned tuna, Swiss cheese, celery, green onions, tomato, lettuce, whole-wheat bread

CHECK FOR: Reduced-fat mayonnaise, white pepper

NUTRITIONAL ANALYSIS PER SERVING (½ SANDWICH): 240 calories, 6 g fat, 2.5 g saturated fat, 28 g protein, 18 g carbohydrates, 2 g fiber, 470 mg sodium

12 ounces canned tuna
2 slices Swiss cheese
1 stalk celery, finely diced
1 tablespoon finely diced green onions
¼ cup reduced-fat mayonnaise
¼ teaspoon ground white pepper
1 tomato, sliced
4 leaves lettuce
4 slices whole-wheat bread

Preheat a panini press. If you don't have a panini press, you can prepare this sandwich the same way you would a grilled cheese sandwich.

Drain the tuna, pressing down to remove all liquid.

In a medium bowl, combine the tuna, celery, green onions, mayonnaise and pepper.

Place a slice of bread in the panini press. Place a slice of cheese on the bread followed by ½ of the tuna mixture and the sliced tomato and lettuce. Add a second slice of bread. Cook until the cheese is melted. Cut the sandwich in half. Repeat with the remaining ingredients.

Grilled vegetable panini

Leftover sun-dried tomato pesto mayo can be stored in the refrigerator for up to one week and used on any type of sandwich or as a vegetable dip.

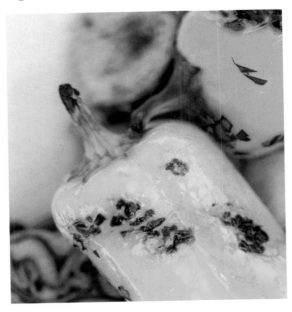

SHOPPING LIST: Sun-dried tomatoes, fresh basil, pumpkin seeds, Parmesan cheese, zucchini, summer squash, red bell pepper, portobello mushrooms, red onion, whole-wheat bread, provolone cheese

CHECK FOR: Olive oil, garlic, lemon juice, kosher salt, reduced-fat mayonnaise, cooking spray

NUTRITIONAL ANALYSIS PER SERVING (½ SANDWICH): 250 calories, 10 g fat, 3 g saturated fat, 11 g protein, 34 g carbohydrates, 3 g fiber, 610 mg sodium

½ cup sun-dried tomatoes, rehydrated in hot water
12 fresh basil leaves
2 tablespoons pumpkin seeds
2 tablespoons Parmesan cheese
1 tablespoon olive oil
1 tablespoon garlic
2 teaspoons lemon juice
¼ teaspoon kosher salt
2 cups reduced-fat mayonnaise
¼ zucchini, cut in planks
¼ summer squash, cut in planks
¼ red bell pepper, cut in planks
¼ cup sliced portobello mushrooms
¼ cup sliced red onion
2 slices whole-wheat bread
1 slice provolone cheese

In a food processor, combine the tomatoes, basil, seeds, cheese, oil, garlic, lemon juice and salt. Process until the ingredients are well blended and somewhat smooth, about 1-2 minutes. Transfer the mixture to a medium-sized bowl, and whisk in the mayonnaise.

Preheat a panini press. Prepare the vegetables. Grill the vegetables, except for the onions; set aside. Preheat a small sauté pan to medium heat; add cooking spray. Sauté the onions until golden and caramelized. Set aside to cool.

Spread ½ tablespoon of sun-dried tomato pesto mayo on each slice of bread. Layer one of the slices with the vegetables and cheese and top with the other slice. Lightly spray the press with cooking spray. Place the sandwich on the press and cook until the cheese is melted.

Tomato, basil and mozzarella hoagie

SERVINGS: 4 | ●◖●

If you're short on time, set the oven to 350 F, but be careful not to let the bread dry out. To cut back on fat, use part-skim mozzarella cheese.

SHOPPING LIST: Hoagie roll or focaccia bread, mozzarella cheese, globe tomatoes (see ingredients on page 219 for basil pesto mayo)

CHECK FOR: Kosher salt, pepper, cooking spray

NUTRITIONAL ANALYSIS PER SERVING (1 SANDWICH): 250 calories, 11 g fat, 3.5 g saturated fat, 12 g protein, 26 g carbohydrates, 1 g fiber, 580 mg sodium

8 (3-inch) pieces light hoagie roll or focaccia bread
4 ounces whole-milk mozzarella cheese, sliced into 4 pieces
4 tablespoons basil pesto mayo (see page 219)
4 globe tomatoes, sliced ½-inch thick
¼ teaspoon kosher salt
¼ teaspoon ground black pepper

Preheat oven to 300 F. Or if you have a panini press, preheat it and spray cooking spray on the top and bottom grills so the sandwiches won't stick.

Spread 1 tablespoon of basil pesto mayo over the hoagie roll or focaccia bread pieces.

Place the tomato slices and mozzarella cheese on four pieces of bread. Season with kosher salt and black pepper.

Top with the remaining pieces of bread. Put the sandwiches on a baking sheet and place in oven. If using a panini press, carefully set sandwiches on the grill and close.

Check the sandwiches at 5 minutes. Remove when they're hot and the cheese is melted. (Once they've cooled, extra sandwiches can be stored in the refrigerator for 1-2 days.)

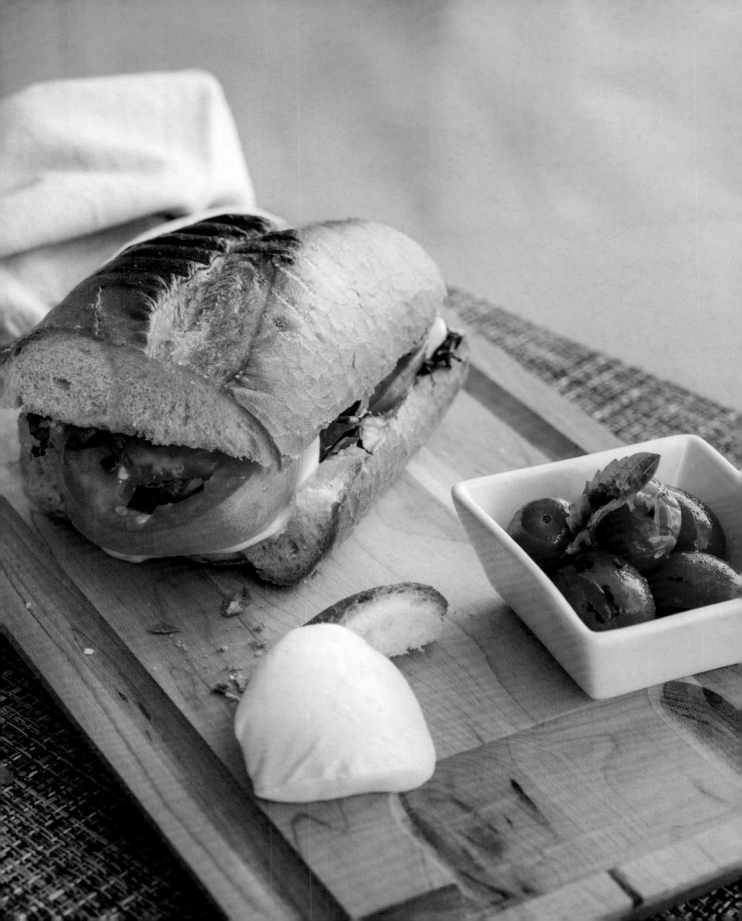

Cobb salad

SERVINGS: 1 | ●● ●●◖

Cobb is a style of a salad, but you can make it your own! Add or substitute other options such as freshly chopped mushrooms, broccoli or bell peppers. You can also try a mixture of different salad greens (spring mix shown). If swapping out the sharp cheddar, make sure to use another flavorful cheese such as feta, blue cheese, goat cheese or aged Parmesan.

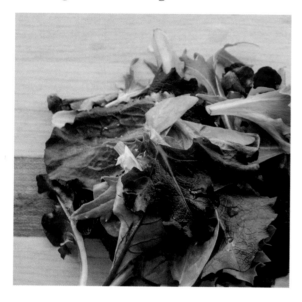

1 head Boston bibb lettuce, or whatever you have on hand, washed and chopped
2 tablespoons bacon or Canadian bacon, cooked crispy and diced
1 hard-boiled medium egg, sliced or quartered
½ cup diced cucumbers
½ cup diced tomatoes
2 ½ tablespoons shredded sharp cheddar cheese
4 ounces grilled chicken breast, sliced

Wash and prepare all ingredients.

Place the lettuce on a serving plate and layer with the bacon, hard-boiled egg, cucumbers, tomatoes and cheese. Top with the grilled chicken breast slices.

Serve with 1 tablespoon of your favorite low-calorie dressing or balsamic vinegar.

SHOPPING LIST: Boston bibb lettuce, bacon or Canadian bacon, cucumber, tomato, sharp cheddar cheese, chicken breast

CHECK FOR: Eggs, dressing

NUTRITIONAL ANALYSIS PER SERVING (1 SALAD): 310 calories, 13 g fat, 5 g saturated fat, 39 g protein, 12 g carbohydrates, 3 g fiber, 420 mg sodium

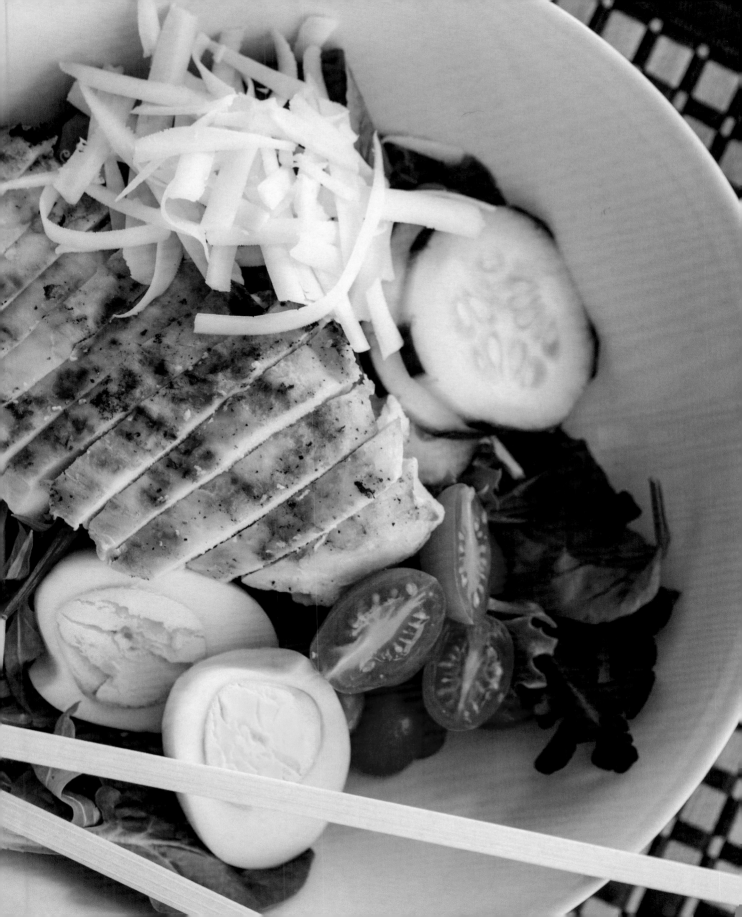

Greek pasta salad

If you'll be eating this throughout the week, keep the dressing separate, and add and toss before eating. This salad can also be made without the noodles, or you can add grilled chicken breast, quinoa, hard-boiled egg or chickpeas (garbanzo beans) for extra protein. For a simplified Greek pasta salad, just add Italian dressing and crumbled feta cheese instead of making your own dressing.

SHOPPING LIST: Hot house cucumber, yellow bell pepper, red onion, celery, Roma tomatoes, romaine lettuce, whole-wheat pasta, feta cheese, Greek olives, cottage cheese, Greek yogurt, Italian dressing, dill weed, fresh oregano, basil or parsley (optional)

CHECK FOR: Pepper

NUTRITIONAL ANALYSIS PER SERVING (¼ SALAD): 190 calories, 6 g fat, 1.5 g saturated fat, 7 g protein, 29 g carbohydrates, 4 g fiber, 370 mg sodium

1 hot house cucumber, diced
1 yellow bell pepper, diced
½ red onion, diced
2 stalks celery, diced
2 Roma tomatoes, diced
1 head romaine lettuce, washed, drained and chopped
2 cups uncooked whole-wheat pasta
¼ cup feta cheese
Greek (Kalamata) olives
Fresh herbs for garnish: oregano, basil or parsley (optional)

DRESSING (MAKES ABOUT 24 SERVINGS)
1 cup 1% cottage cheese
1 cup plain Greek yogurt
1 cup fat-free Italian dressing
½ cup feta cheese
1 teaspoon dry dill weed
¼ teaspoon ground black pepper

Cook the pasta according to the package directions and drain. Rinse under cool water, drain, lightly toss with olive oil and chill.

Prepare all the vegetables, if not yet diced. Combine all ingredients for the dressing in a food processor.

Combine the salad ingredients: Mix the pasta, lettuce, vegetables and ½ cup of the dressing in a large bowl. Add the feta cheese.

Garnish with fresh chopped oregano, basil or parsley or other fresh herbs, and place a Greek olive on top.

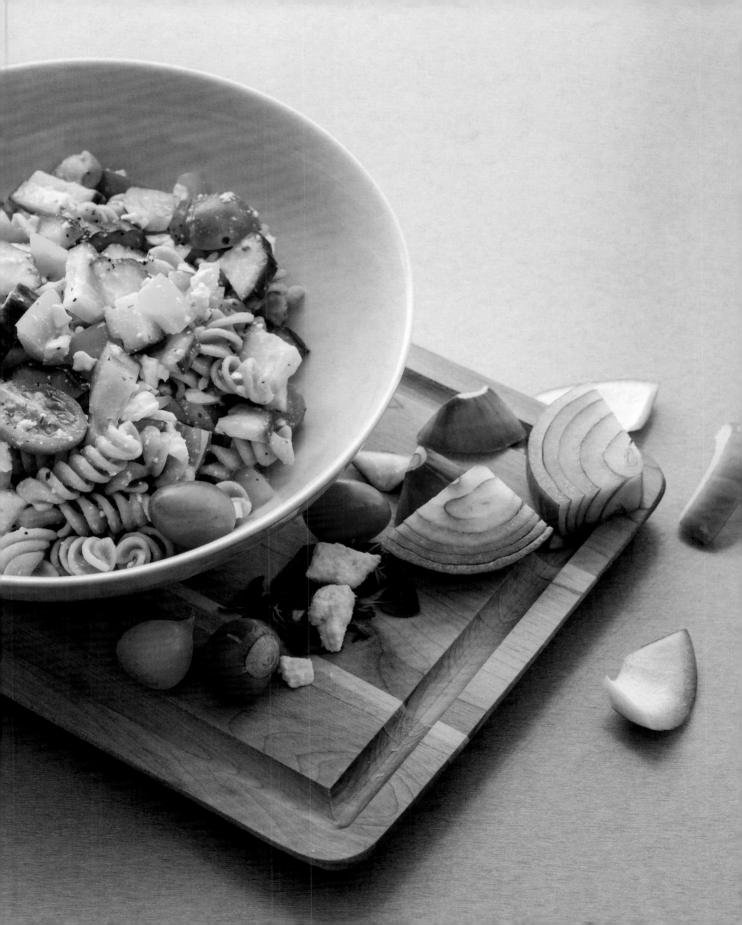

Mix-and-match salads

Use the chart below to create fun and healthy salads. Assemble your salad by picking one or more ingredients from each column. To get the best flavor out of your salad, toss it with 2 tablespoons of dressing so that each ingredient is lightly covered with flavor.

Be adventurous and experiment. Baby kale can be mixed in with romaine lettuce to make an even more nutritional Caesar salad. Another option is to add up to ½ cup of fresh fruit. If you're taking a salad to work, keep the dressing separate until you're ready to eat.

TRY 1 OF THESE GREENS (2 CUPS)	WITH 1 OF THESE VEGGIES (½ CUP)	PLUS 1 OF THESE PROTEINS (3 OUNCES/ ½ CUP)	PLUS 1 OF THESE TOPPINGS (2 TABLESPOONS)	AND 1 OF THESE DRESSINGS (2 TABLESPOONS)
Arugula	Artichokes	Black beans	Croutons	Balsamic vinegar
Baby kale	Beets	Chicken breast	Dried fruit	Cilantro lime
Bibb lettuce	Bell peppers	Chickpeas	Fresh fruit	Light Caesar
Cabbage	Broccoli	Edamame	Hard or sharp cheese	Light Italian
Leaf lettuce	Carrots	Hard-boiled eggs	Nuts	Low-fat ranch
Romaine	Cauliflower	Kidney beans	Seeds	Low-fat raspberry vinaigrette
Spinach	Cucumbers	Lean ground beef		Olive oil
Spring mix	Mushrooms	Salmon		Other vinegars
	Onions	Shrimp		Salsa or taco sauce
	Peas	Tofu (firm)		
	Radishes	Turkey breast		
	Tomatoes			

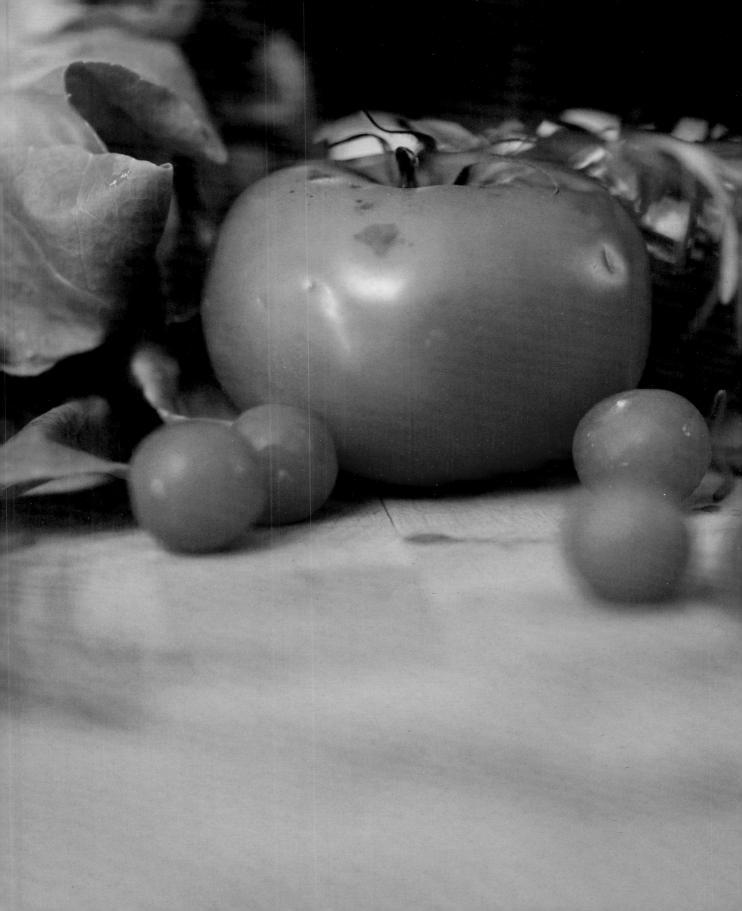

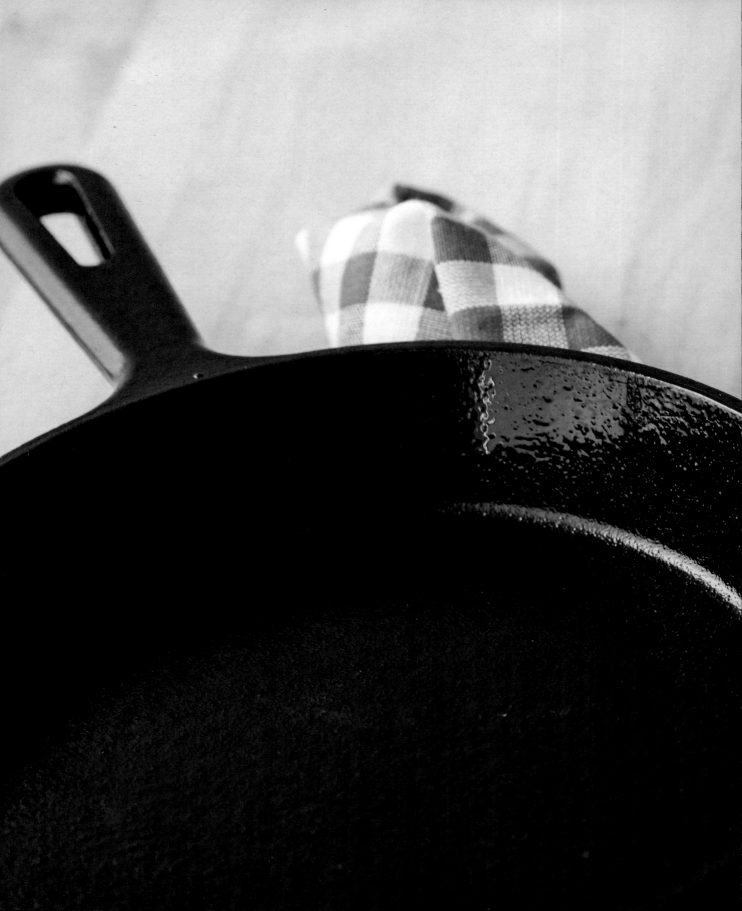

Soups

Cuban black bean soup

You can choose to purée all the beans in this soup, a portion of them (as in this recipe) or none. If you add less stock at the end — about half of what's called for — you can serve this as a thicker purée for tacos, dip, or as a spread on a tostada.

¾ cup dried black beans, rinsed and soaked
    overnight, or 2 cups cooked black beans*
1 bay leaf
½ onion, diced
2 celery stalks, diced
1 carrot, diced
2 cups water (or vegetable or chicken stock)
2 tablespoons orange juice concentrate
2 teaspoons ground cumin
1 tablespoon fresh oregano
1 ½ teaspoon sea salt
½ teaspoon minced garlic

Lightly coat a soup pot with cooking spray. Over medium heat, sauté onions, celery and carrots approximately 5 minutes.

Add the beans, bay leaf, and water or stock and simmer until the beans are very soft. This will take approximately 25-30 minutes, provided the beans were soaked overnight.

When the beans are cooked, pour ¾ of the mixture into a blender or mixing bowl and purée until smooth and thick.

Return puréed mixture to soup pot and season with orange juice concentrate, cumin, oregano and salt. Stir in minced garlic and the remaining liquid until reaching the consistency you desire.

* To make this recipe with canned beans, use 2 cans black beans, rinsed. Boil the vegetables in 1-2 cups water for 10 minutes. Blend in the black beans and 1 cup of stock, and purée until thick. Continue with the last step.

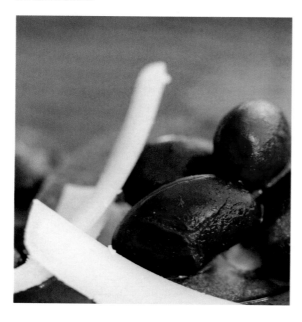

SHOPPING LIST: Black beans, bay leaves, onion, celery, carrot, orange juice concentrate, fresh oregano, vegetable or chicken stock (optional)

CHECK FOR: Cumin, sea salt, garlic, cooking spray

NUTRITIONAL ANALYSIS PER SERVING (1 CUP): 200 calories, 5 g fat, 1 g saturated fat, 11 g protein, 29 g carbohydrates, 10 g fiber, 460 mg sodium

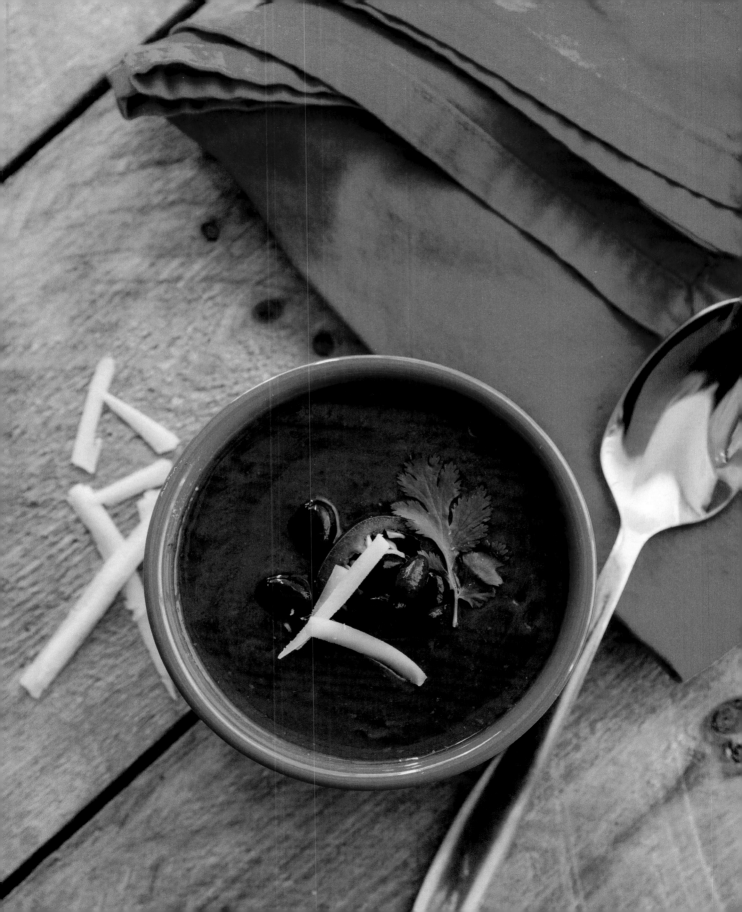

Creamy butternut squash soup

SERVINGS: 6 |

The brown sugar in the recipe helps pull out the sweet undertones of the butternut squash. If you prefer a savory flavor, swap out the cinnamon, nutmeg and clove, and add chopped fresh sage or thyme near the end of the cooking.

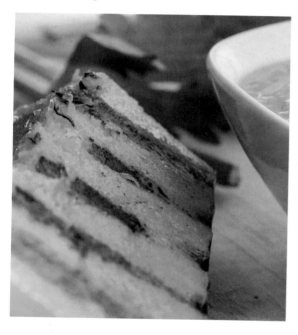

SHOPPING LIST: Butternut squash, onion, carrots, celery, vegetable broth, half-and-half

CHECK FOR: Olive oil, brown sugar, nutmeg, cinnamon, kosher salt, cornstarch

NUTRITIONAL ANALYSIS PER SERVING (1 CUP): 130 calories, 1.5 g fat, .5 g saturated fat, 2 g protein, 28 g carbohydrates, 3 g fiber, 370 mg sodium

4 cups roasted butternut squash
1 teaspoon olive oil
2 cups chopped onions
1 cup chopped carrots
1 cup chopped celery
1 cup vegetable broth
2 cups water
3 tablespoons brown sugar
¼ teaspoon nutmeg
½ teaspoon cinnamon
¾ teaspoon kosher salt
¼ cup cornstarch
¼ cup water
¼ cup half-and-half

Preheat oven to 400 F. Cut butternut squash in half, remove the seeds and lay skin-side up in a baking pan. Add 4 cups water to the pan. Roast 30-45 minutes until fork easily pierces squash.

Heat a large soup pot to medium-high heat. Add the olive oil, followed by the chopped vegetables. Sauté 5-10 minutes until soft and tender. (You may need to reduce the heat.)

Add vegetable broth, 2 cups water, brown sugar, nutmeg, cinnamon and salt. Let soup simmer about 15 minutes. Add the roasted squash. Remove from heat and let cool slightly. Transfer small amounts at a time to a blender. Purée the entire batch of soup.

Return mixture to the soup pot and bring to a boil. Mix together the cornstarch and ¼ cup water and slowly add (about 1 tablespoon at a time) to the boiling soup, whisking until thickened. When desired consistency is achieved, add the half-and-half and serve.

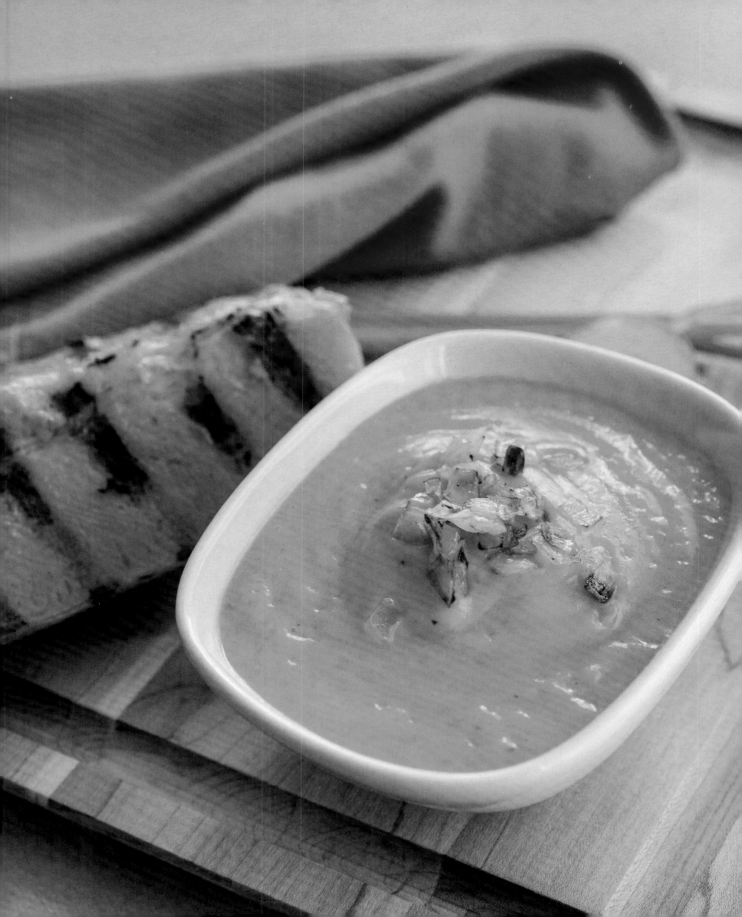

Broccoli cheddar soup

SERVINGS: 8 | ● ● ◖

It's best to purchase a block of cheddar cheese and shred your own. Pre-shredded cheeses contain cellulose powder to keep the cheese from sticking together. Pre-shredded cheese may not melt as well as cheese you shred yourself.

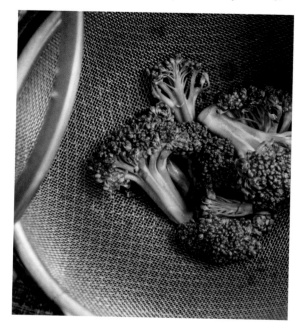

SHOPPING LIST: Onion, broccoli, vegetable stock or broth, cream cheese, cornstarch or arrowroot, half-and-half, sharp cheddar cheese

CHECK FOR: Onion powder, garlic powder, salt, pepper

NUTRITIONAL ANALYSIS PER SERVING
(1 CUP): 180 calories, 10 g fat, 7 g saturated fat, 9 g protein, 14 g carbohydrates, 2 g fiber, 490 mg sodium

1 onion, finely chopped
2 heads of broccoli, rinsed and cut into florets
6 cups vegetable stock (or broccoli broth)
1 tablespoon onion powder
1 teaspoon garlic powder
1 teaspoon salt
6 tablespoons low-fat cream cheese
2 tablespoons cornstarch (or arrowroot),
    mixed with 2 tablespoons cold water
1 cup half-and-half
¾ cup shredded 2% milk sharp cheddar cheese
Ground black pepper to taste

Heat a soup pot to medium-high heat. Add onion and sauté until translucent.

Add the vegetable stock, onion and garlic powder and salt. Bring the stock to a simmer. Add the broccoli florets and let simmer for 10-15 minutes until the broccoli is tender.

Remove from heat and let cool slightly. Add the cream cheese. (It will be lumpy.) Transfer the soup in batches to a food processor or blender and process until smooth. You can also use an immersion blender if you have one.

Return the blended mixture to the soup pot and place it over medium heat. When soup begins to simmer, slowly add the cornstarch or arrowroot mixed with water. Soup will thicken in about a minute.

When thick, add the half-and-half, which will give the soup its creamy color. Turn off the heat and add the cheese. Whisk until the cheese is well blended. Add ground pepper to taste and serve.

Vegetable lentil soup

Many types of lentils can be used in this soup, such as red lentils, to change the color. The soup is also great puréed.

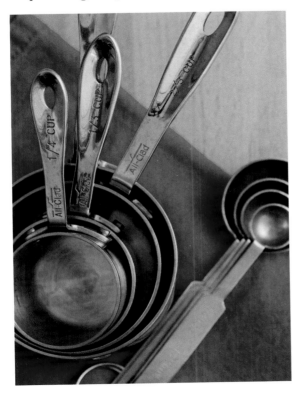

1 ½ cups uncooked lentils
1 tablespoon olive oil
3 cups diced carrots
2 cups diced onions
1 ½ cups diced celery
10 cups water or vegetable stock
2 lemons, juiced
1 bay leaf
1 teaspoon kosher salt
¼ teaspoon ground black pepper

Partially cook lentils in a steamer basket for approximately 20 minutes. Drain and set aside.

Add the olive oil to a medium to large soup pot. Heat the oil and add the diced carrots, onions and celery. Cook for approximately 5 minutes at medium heat, stirring frequently. Add the water or vegetable stock and bring to a boil.

Add the partially cooked lentils, lemon juice, bay leaf, salt and pepper and bring to a boil. Let simmer for approximately 15 minutes.

Remove the bay leaf. Taste the soup and adjust the seasoning, if needed, before serving.

SHOPPING LIST: Lentils, carrots, onion, celery, lemons, vegetable stock (optional)

CHECK FOR: Olive oil, bay leaves, kosher salt, pepper

NUTRITIONAL ANALYSIS PER SERVING
(1 CUP): 150 calories, 1 g fat, 8 g protein,
26 g carbohydrates, 8 g fiber, 340 mg sodium

White bean and kale soup

SERVINGS: 12 |

If you're looking for a hearty winter soup, add kielbasa sausage to this recipe. Chop the sausage into small pieces to reduce calories. Add it early while sautéing the vegetables to release its flavor.

SHOPPING LIST: White beans, kale, onion, carrots, fresh thyme, fresh rosemary, white wine, vegetable stock

CHECK FOR: Olive oil, bay leaves, kosher salt, pepper

NUTRITIONAL ANALYSIS PER SERVING (½ CUP): 130 calories, 1.5 g fat, 6 g protein, 21 g carbohydrates, 8 g fiber, 420 mg sodium

3 cups cooked white beans (2 cans or 1 cup dry)
12 cups cleaned and chopped kale
2 cups chopped onions
2 cups chopped carrots
2 teaspoons chopped fresh thyme
1 teaspoon chopped fresh rosemary
1 tablespoon olive oil
1 cup white wine
10 cups vegetable stock
1 bay leaf
1 teaspoon kosher salt
¼ teaspoon ground black pepper

If using dried white beans, prepare the dried beans according to package directions. If using canned beans, rinse the beans.

Heat a large soup pot to medium heat. Add the oil, onions and carrots and cook for 5 minutes. Add the kale and the wine. Let simmer until the liquid reduces by half.

Add the thyme, rosemary, vegetable stock, bay leaf, salt and pepper and bring to a boil. Add the beans, reduce heat and let simmer for 20 minutes. Remove the bay leaf before serving.

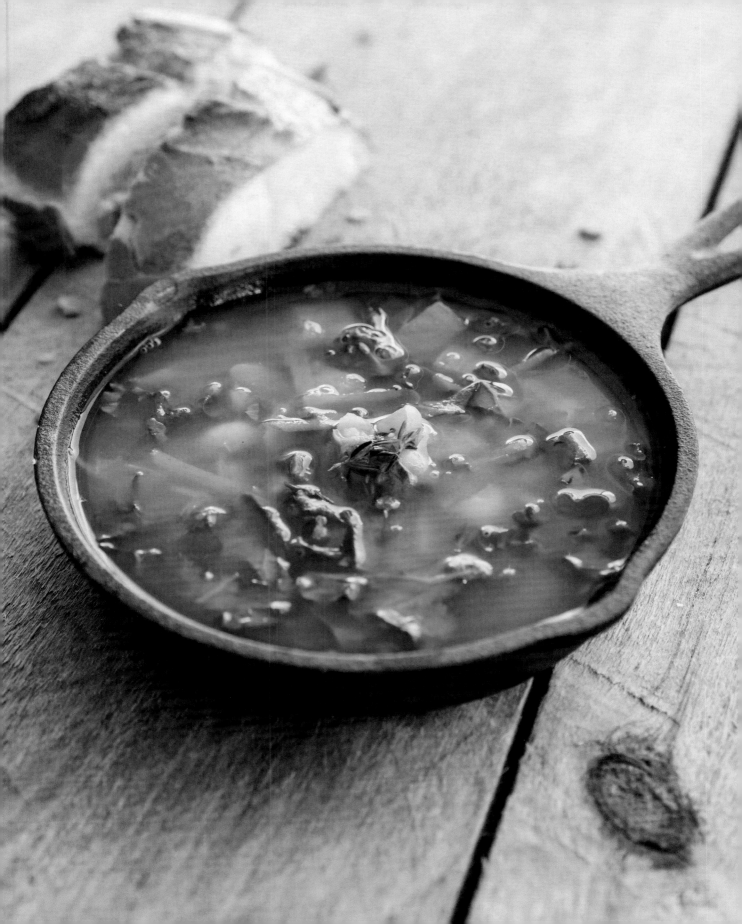

Turkey wild rice chowder

Instead of using cornstarch, another way to thicken this soup and give it a creamy texture is to whisk in leftover mashed potatoes, mashed turnips or mashed cauliflower. Using half-and-half in place of skim milk will also create a creamier soup — just keep in mind it will also increase calories and fat.

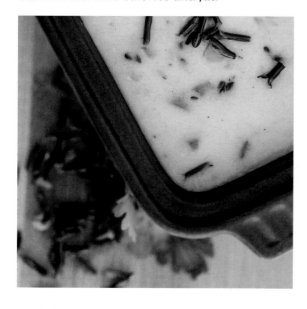

SHOPPING LIST: Low-sodium chicken stock, carrots, onion, celery, turkey breast, wild rice, fresh rosemary, fresh thyme

CHECK FOR: Skim milk, salt, pepper, cornstarch or arrowroot

NUTRITIONAL ANALYSIS PER SERVING (1 CUP): 170 calories, 3 g fat, 1.5 g saturated fat, 20 g protein, 15 g carbohydrates, 2 g fiber, 350 mg sodium

6 cups low-sodium chicken stock
1 carrot, chopped
1 onion, finely diced
3 celery stalks, chopped
8 ounces cooked turkey breast, cut into medium-sized chunks
1 cup cooked wild rice
1 cup skim milk
1 tablespoon chopped fresh rosemary
1 tablespoon chopped fresh thyme
1 teaspoon salt
¼ teaspoon ground black pepper
2 tablespoons cornstarch or arrowroot
2 tablespoons cold water

Follow package directions to cook the wild rice: ¼ cup raw rice equals about 1 cup cooked.

Heat a medium to large soup pot. Add the carrots, onion and celery to the warm pot, and stir until vegetables are tender.

Add the chicken stock. Let it simmer and reduce down to approximately 4 cups. Add the fresh rosemary and thyme, salt, pepper, chopped turkey and wild rice. Taste the soup to check the seasonings, and adjust if needed. Add the skim milk, and let soup return to a low boil.

Mix the cornstarch or arrowroot with the water. Once the soup has reached a low boil, whisk in the mixture, stirring until the soup thickens to chowder consistency.

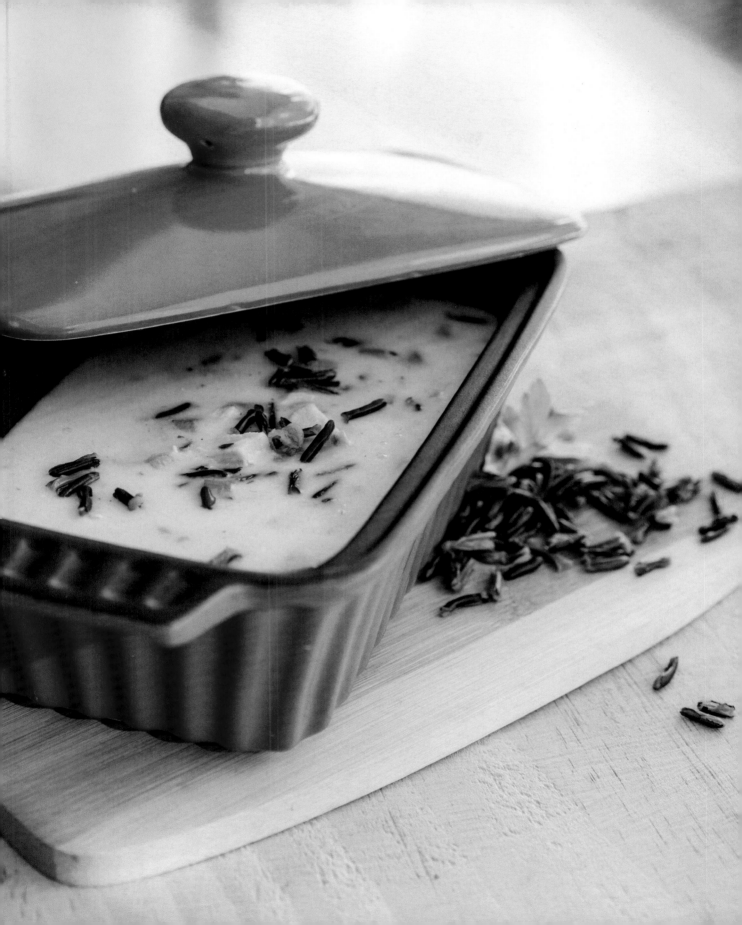

Minestrone soup

This soup is a great way to use leftover vegetables you have in the refrigerator — such as grilled vegetables, bell peppers, green beans or baby carrots — before they go bad.

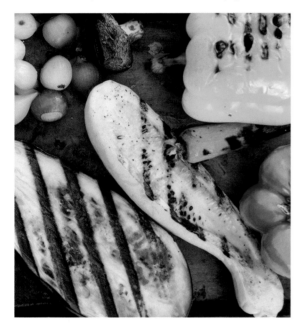

SHOPPING LIST: Sweet onion, celery, carrots, low-sodium vegetable or chicken broth, low-sodium stewed tomatoes, low-sodium V8 juice, cannellini beans, whole-wheat elbow or shells pasta, zucchini

CHECK FOR: Olive oil, garlic, basil, oregano, thyme, salt, pepper

NUTRITIONAL ANALYSIS PER SERVING (½ CUP): 130 calories, 1 g fat, 6 g protein, 25 g carbohydrates, 7 g fiber, 370 mg sodium

¼ teaspoon olive oil
1 cup chopped sweet onion
½ cup chopped celery
½ cup diced carrots
2 cloves garlic, minced
3 cups low-sodium vegetable or chicken broth
3 cups water
1 14.5-ounce can low-sodium stewed toma-
    toes, not drained
1 small can low-sodium V8 juice
1 14.5-ounce can cannellini beans, drained
    and rinsed
1 cup cooked whole-wheat pasta, shells or elbow
1 cup chopped zucchini
1 tablespoon dry basil
1 tablespoon dry oregano
2 teaspoons dry thyme
1 teaspoon salt
¼ teaspoon ground black pepper

Heat a medium to large soup pot to medium-high heat. Add the olive oil, onion, celery and carrots and sauté approximately 3-4 minutes until softened.

Add the garlic and continue to sauté for 1 minute, taking care not to let it burn. Add the dried herbs and salt and pepper.

Add the zucchini, tomatoes, broth, V8 juice and water. Bring to a boil over high heat. Reduce heat, add cannellini beans and simmer for 15 minutes. Add the cooked pasta and simmer 5 more minutes.

Taste for flavor before serving. It takes time for dry herbs and spices to release their flavor, so don't taste too soon after adding them.

Three bean chili

SERVINGS: 12 |

To reduce the sodium in this recipe, purchase low-sodium canned beans or make sure to rinse the beans before adding them to the soup.

SHOPPING LIST: Onion, poblano peppers, ground beef, pinto beans, navy beans, black beans, limes, Tabasco, low-sodium diced tomatoes, unsalted vegetable stock, fresh cilantro

CHECK FOR: Olive or canola oil, garlic, chili powder, cumin, kosher salt

NUTRITIONAL ANALYSIS PER SERVING (½ CUP): 190 calories, 2.5 g fat, 1 g saturated fat, 16 g protein, 28 g carbohydrates, 8 g fiber, 160 mg sodium

1 teaspoon olive or canola oil
1 white onion, diced
1 tablespoon minced garlic
2 poblano peppers, seeded and diced
1 pound lean ground beef
1 can pinto beans, rinsed
1 can navy beans, rinsed
1 can black beans, rinsed
3 cans low-sodium diced tomatoes
2 cups unsalted vegetable stock
1 tablespoon chili powder
1 teaspoon ground cumin
1 teaspoon kosher salt
1 teaspoon Tabasco
2 limes, freshly squeezed
¼ cup chopped fresh cilantro

Heat a large soup pot over medium heat. Once warm, add the oil, onions, garlic and poblano peppers to the pot and sauté about 2-4 minutes until they start to soften.

Add the ground beef and cook until it's fully browned. Then add the beans, diced tomatoes, vegetable stock, spices, Tabasco, and freshly squeezed lime juice. Simmer approximately 20 minutes. Taste and adjust the spices if needed.

Garnish each bowl with fresh cilantro and serve immediately.

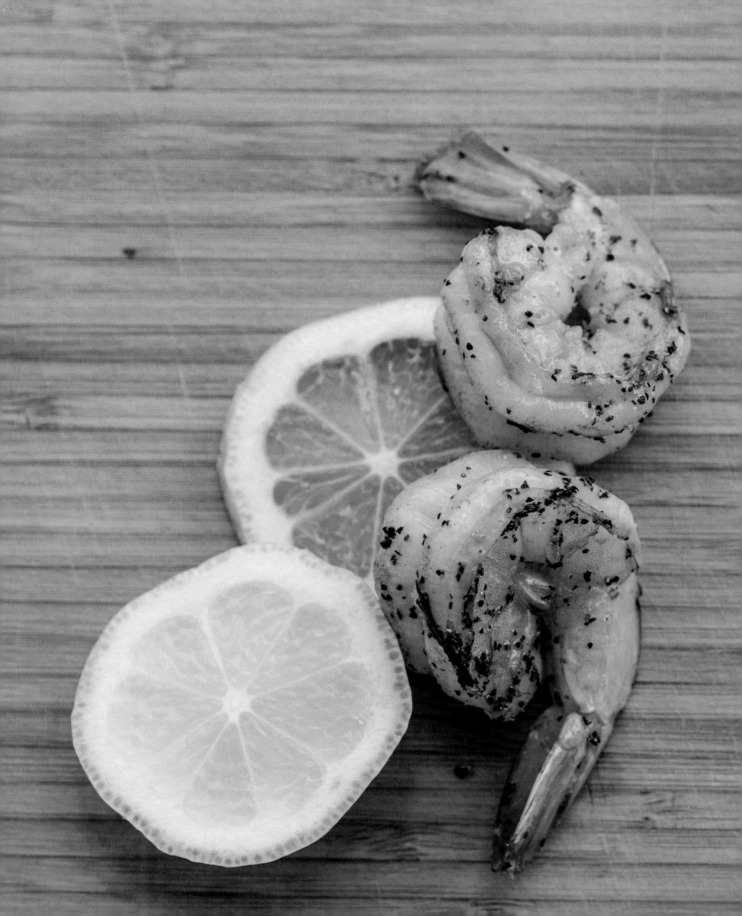

Appetizers & snacks

Black bean and corn salsa

SERVINGS: 6 |

*Add this salsa to your favorite Mexican dish.
It goes well with chicken, fish, pork or beef.*

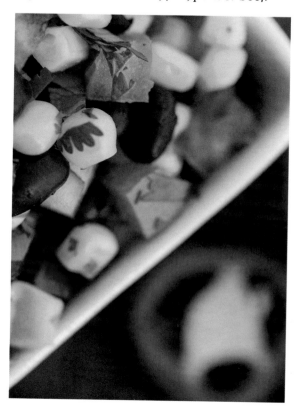

2 Roma tomatoes, seeded and diced
¼ cup minced red onion
¼ cup chopped red bell pepper
½ cup black beans
¼ cup corn
1 tablespoon chopped fresh cilantro
1 tablespoon minced garlic
1 tablespoon lime juice
½ teaspoon ground cumin
¼ teaspoon salt

In a medium bowl, combine the tomatoes,
onion, pepper, beans and corn. In a separate
bowl, mix together the cilantro, garlic, lime
juice, cumin and salt and add to the bean-
corn mixture.

Taste for flavor. Add additional seasonings
if desired.

SHOPPING LIST: Roma tomatoes, onion,
red bell pepper, fresh cilantro, black beans,
corn, lime juice

CHECK FOR: Garlic, cumin, salt

NUTRITIONAL ANALYSIS PER SERVING (⅓
CUP): 40 calories, 2 g protein, 9 g carbohydrates,
2 g fiber, 85 mg sodium

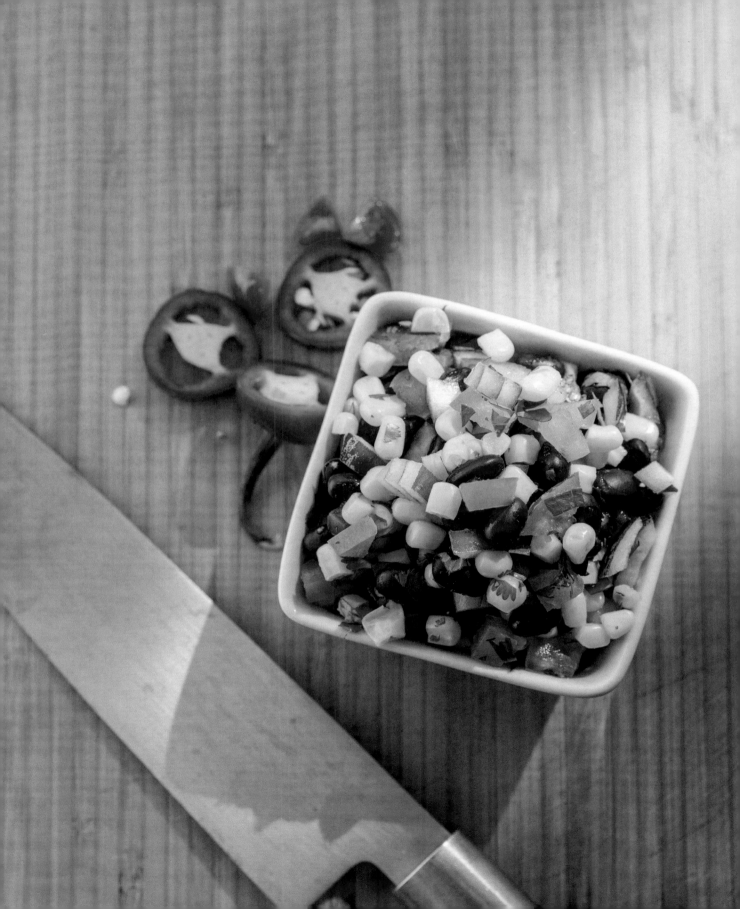

Roasted red pepper hummus

SERVINGS: 16

Using roasted red peppers from a can or a jar works just as well. However, make sure they're packed in water and not oil. You can add more nutrition and flavor by adding fresh or pickled jalapenos, roasted poblanos, carrots, red onion and cilantro. This hummus is perfect for a midafternoon snack with veggies or baked pita chips. You can also use it as a spread on sandwiches and wraps.

SHOPPING LIST: Red bell peppers, chickpeas, white sesame seeds, lemon juice, fresh parsley

CHECK FOR: Olive oil, cumin, onion powder, garlic powder, kosher salt, cayenne pepper

NUTRITIONAL ANALYSIS PER SERVING (3 TABLESPOONS): 45 calories, 2 g fat, 2 g protein, 6 g carbohydrates, 2 g fiber, 160 mg sodium

2 large or 3 medium red bell peppers
2 cups chickpeas (garbanzo beans), drained and rinsed
2 tablespoons white sesame seeds
1 tablespoon lemon juice
1 tablespoon olive oil
¼ cup fresh parsley
1 ¼ teaspoon ground cumin
1 teaspoon onion powder
1 teaspoon garlic powder
1 teaspoon kosher salt
¼ teaspoon cayenne pepper

Roast the red bell peppers on a grill or in an oven at medium heat until the skin turns dark brown or black on all sides. Remove the skin and the seeds from the peppers and rinse the peppers.

In a food processor, add 1 cup roasted red pepper and the remaining ingredients. Process until the mixture is smooth. Transfer to a dish and serve.

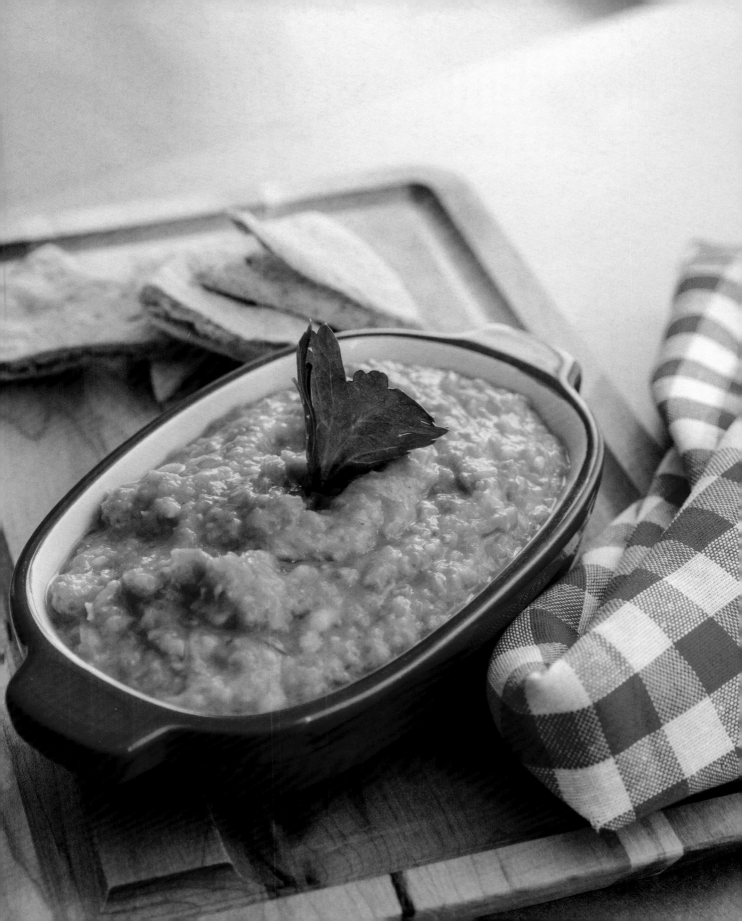

Spinach artichoke dip

SERVINGS: 8 |

You can use baby kale in this recipe instead of baby spinach. For a more peppery flavor, replace a small amount of the spinach with arugula.

SHOPPING LIST: Baby spinach, artichokes, shallots or green onions, fat-free cream cheese, Parmesan cheese

CHECK FOR: Garlic, olive oil, skim milk

NUTRITIONAL ANALYSIS PER SERVING (¼ CUP): 110 calories, 5 g fat, 3 g saturated fat, 7 g protein, 11 g carbohydrates, 4 g fiber, 230 mg sodium

10 cups baby spinach, cleaned and chopped
½ cup minced shallots or green onions
2 teaspoons minced garlic
2 cups canned artichokes
1 teaspoon olive oil
4 ounces fat-free cream cheese
½ cup skim milk
½ cup shredded Parmesan cheese

Drain and quarter the artichokes.

Heat a large nonstick sauté pan to medium heat; add oil. Sauté shallots and garlic until soft. Add the spinach and stir until wilted.

Reduce heat and stir in the artichokes, cream cheese and milk. Whisk until smooth. Add the Parmesan cheese, stirring constantly until the cheese is melted and well-blended. Serve warm with whole-wheat pita chips.

Tomato bruschetta

The tomato mixture in bruschetta also works great as a topping on pasta dishes or with seared chicken breasts and fish.

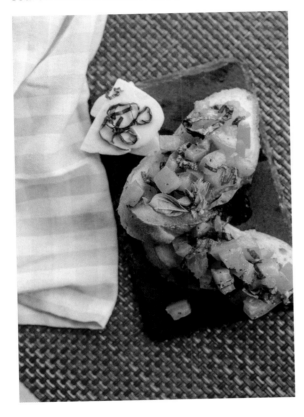

6 Roma tomatoes, seeded and diced
2 tablespoons chopped fresh basil
1 tablespoon minced garlic
Small whole-wheat baguette
1 teaspoon olive oil
¼ teaspoon sea salt
Pinch of ground black pepper

In a small bowl, combine all of the ingredients, except for the baguette. Set aside for 1 hour.

Slice the baguette. Place 4 slices in an oven or toaster oven and toast until slightly golden. To serve, place the tomato mixture on top of the baguette slices.

SHOPPING LIST: Roma tomatoes, fresh basil, whole-wheat baguette

CHECK FOR: Garlic, olive oil, sea salt, pepper

NUTRITIONAL ANALYSIS PER SERVING (1 PIECE): 70 calories, 2 g fat, 2 g protein, 11 g carbohydrates, 1 g fiber, 200 mg sodium

Coconut shrimp

For a darker crust, sauté the coated shrimp in a medium pan with canola oil.

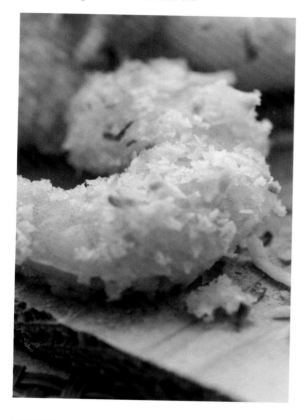

¼ cup sweetened coconut
¼ cup panko breadcrumbs
½ teaspoon kosher salt
½ cup coconut milk
12 large peeled and deveined shrimp

Preheat oven to 375 F. Lightly coat a baking sheet with cooking spray.

Place the coconut, panko and salt in a food processor and process until the mixture is an even consistency. Transfer the mixture to a small bowl. Pour coconut milk into another small bowl.

Arrange in this order: shrimp, coconut milk, panko-coconut mixture, and a baking sheet. Take a shrimp, dip it in the coconut milk, coat with the panko-coconut mixture and place it on the baking sheet. Repeat the process with all of the shrimp. Lightly coat the top of the shrimp with cooking spray.

Bake 10-15 minutes until golden brown.

SHOPPING LIST: Sweetened coconut, panko, coconut milk, large peeled and deveined shrimp

CHECK FOR: Kosher salt, cooking spray

NUTRITIONAL ANALYSIS PER SERVING (2 SHRIMP): 50 calories, 2 g fat, 1.5 g saturated fat, 2 g protein, 7 g carbohydrates, 1 g fiber, 250 mg sodium

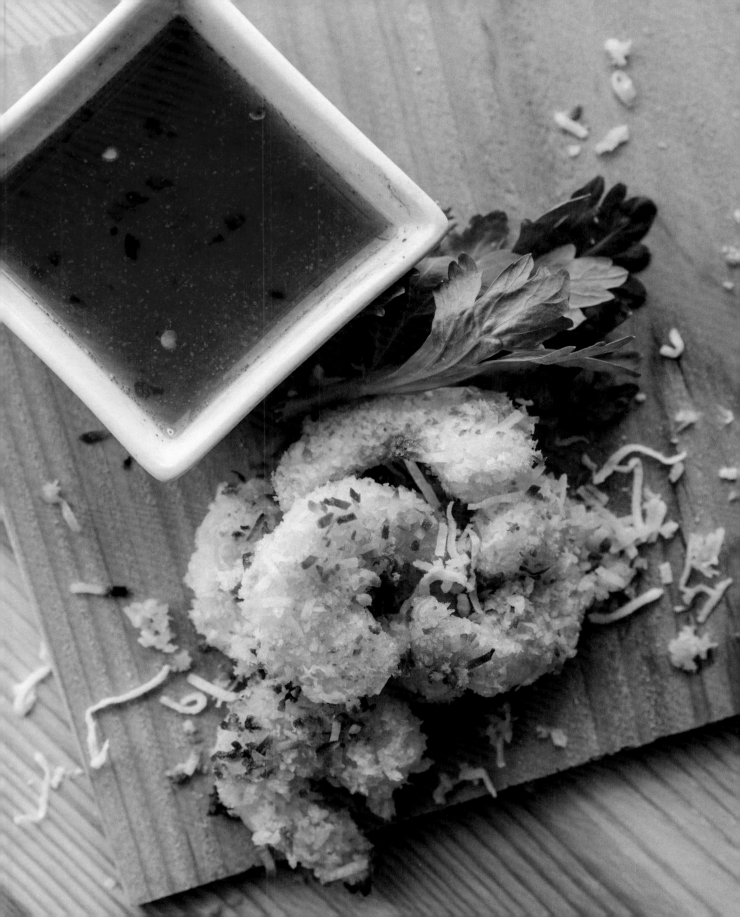

Thai chicken satay

Different thicknesses of meat will determine the length of cooking necessary to reach a minimum temperature of 165 F.

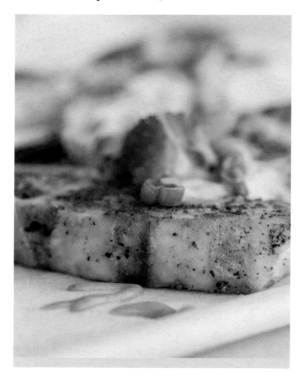

SHOPPING LIST: Wood skewers, chicken breasts, sesame oil, rice wine vinegar, scallions

CHECK FOR: Brown sugar, soy sauce, red pepper flakes, ginger powder, kosher salt, cooking spray

NUTRITIONAL ANALYSIS PER SERVING (1 SKEWER): 320 calories, 6 g fat, 0.5 g saturated fat, 33 g protein, 36 g carbohydrates, 4 g fiber, 780 mg sodium

8 ounces boneless, skinless chicken breasts, trimmed and cut into 1-ounce portions
1 tablespoon sesame oil
2 tablespoon brown sugar
1 tablespoon rice wine vinegar
5 tablespoons soy sauce
2 tablespoon minced scallions
Pinch red pepper flakes
1 teaspoon ginger powder
¼ teaspoon kosher salt

Preheat a grill, cast iron skillet or sauté pan. Prepare the chicken. Soak 2 wood skewers for at least 20 minutes.

Mix the remaining ingredients in a bowl to make the marinade. Place the chicken pieces into the mixture and marinate for about 15 minutes.

When the chicken is finished marinating, thread the chicken pieces onto the skewers. Lightly spray the grill, skillet or sauté pan with cooking spray.

Once the heat source is hot, place the skewers on the cooking surface. If you're grilling or using a cast iron skillet with ridges, cook for approximately 1-2 minutes on each side, depending on the thickness of the meat. If you're using a sauté pan, lightly sear on each side approximately 2 minutes. Cook the chicken to an internal temperature of 165 F.

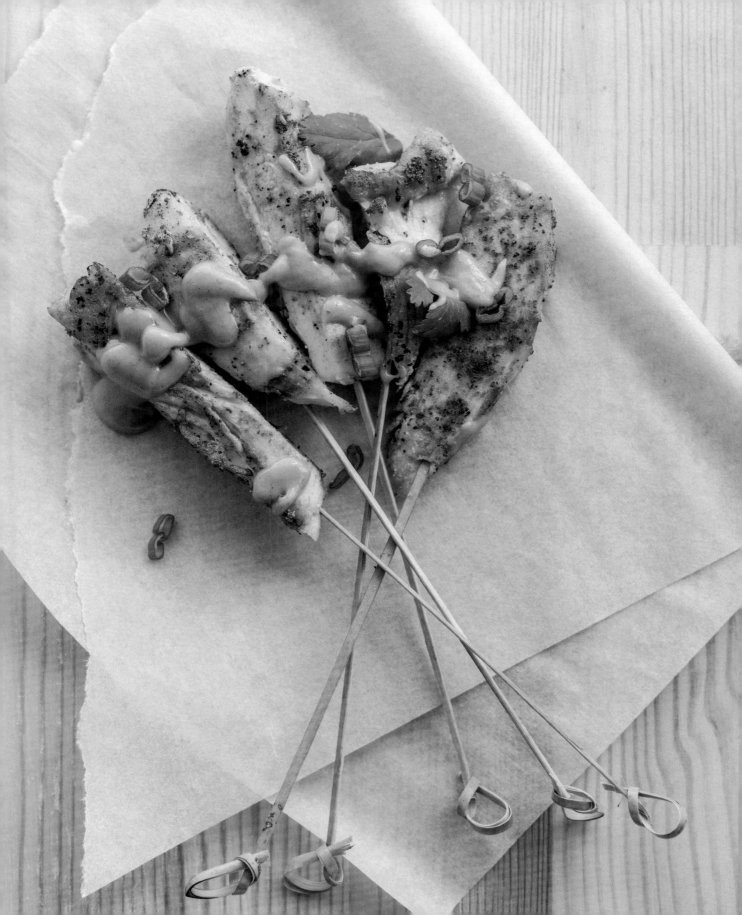

Pesto stuffed mushrooms

SERVINGS: 20

Save the remaining pesto filling for sauces. You can also add light mayonnaise to it and use it as a sandwich spread. If you have a lot of fresh basil in your garden, make a large batch of pesto filling and freeze it.

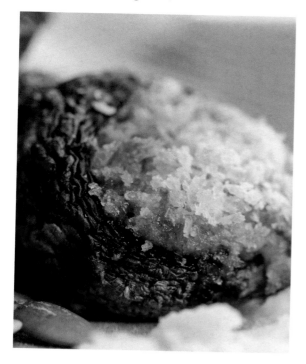

SHOPPING LIST: Panko, fresh parsley, cremini mushrooms, fresh basil, fresh Parmesan cheese, pumpkin seeds, lemon juice

CHECK FOR: Butter, olive oil, garlic, kosher salt

NUTRITIONAL ANALYSIS PER SERVING (1 MUSHROOM): 80 calories, 4 g fat, 3 g protein, 9 g carbohydrates, 1 g fiber, 85 mg sodium

¼ cup butter
1 ½ cups panko breadcrumbs
3 tablespoons chopped fresh parsley
20 cremini mushrooms

PESTO FILLING
2 cups chopped fresh basil leaves
¼ cup shredded Parmesan cheese
2 tablespoons pumpkin seeds
1 tablespoon olive oil
1 tablespoon minced garlic
2 teaspoons lemon juice
½ teaspoon kosher salt

Preheat oven to 350 F. Melt the butter. In a large bowl, combine panko, melted butter and chopped parsley; set aside.

Wash the mushrooms and remove the stems. Line the mushroom caps upside down on a baking sheet.

Prepare a food processor with the S-shaped blade. Place all filling ingredients in the food processor and process until evenly mixed.

Generously stuff each mushroom with the filling mixture. Sprinkle approximately 1 teaspoon of the breadcrumb mixture on top of each filled mushroom. Pat down so the topping sticks to the mushrooms.

Place mushrooms in oven and bake 10-15 minutes until filling and topping are golden brown.

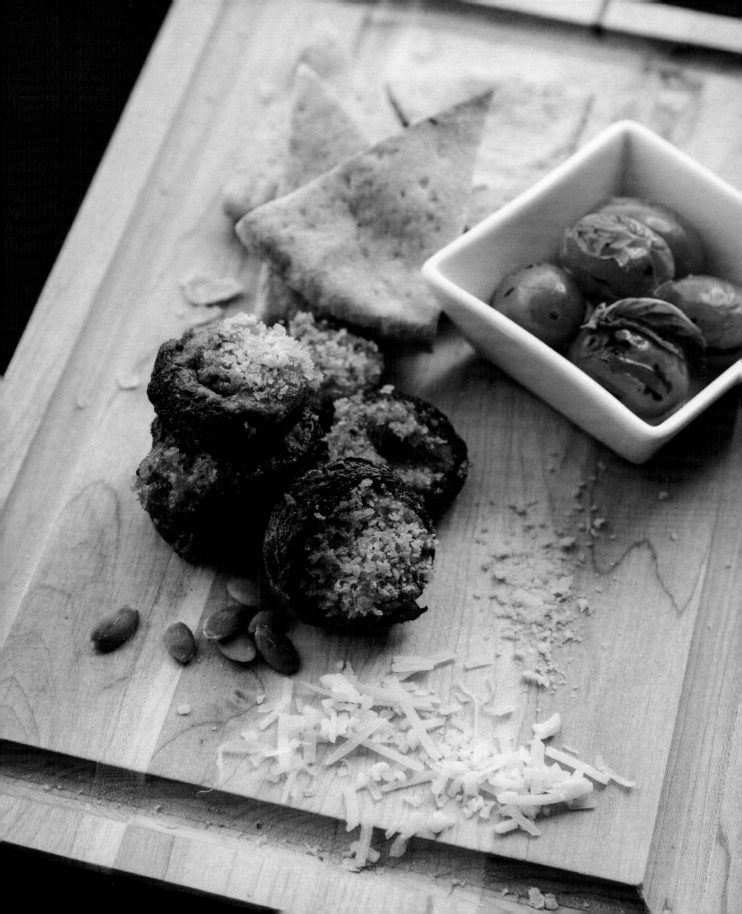

Buffalo zucchini sticks

SERVINGS: 6 |

Try this recipe with other vegetables, such as summer squash or eggplant! For the best success, make sure the panko is ground smaller, so it will stick to the vegetable.

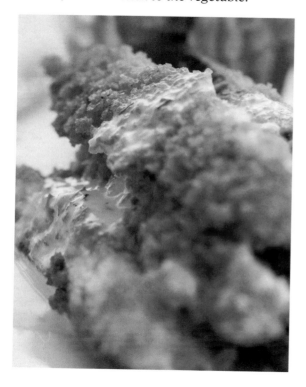

1 cup panko breadcrumbs, ground fine
½ teaspoon salt
½ teaspoon garlic powder
½ teaspoon onion powder
1 egg
2 zucchinis, cut into sticks (planks)
½ cup buffalo sauce

Preheat oven to 425 F. Lightly spray a baking sheet with cooking spray.

In a medium bowl mix the ground panko, salt, garlic powder and onion powder. In a separate bowl, whisk the egg and set aside.

Dip each zucchini stick into the egg mixture, shake off excess egg and dredge into the panko mixture. (Try to keep one hand as the "wet" hand one as the "dry" hand.) Place breaded sticks on the baking sheet, allowing enough space between each one. Repeat until all sticks are coated.

Bake approximately 20-25 minutes or until zucchini is cooked and outside is slightly crunchy.

Dip each stick in bowl of buffalo sauce or drizzle sauce over the top. Serve with a low-fat dip.

SHOPPING LIST: Panko, zucchini, buffalo sauce

CHECK FOR: Salt, garlic powder, onion powder, eggs, cooking spray

NUTRITIONAL ANALYSIS PER SERVING (APPROX. 3 STICKS): 100 calories, 5 g fat, 2 g protein, 12 g carbohydrates, 1 g fiber, 320 mg sodium

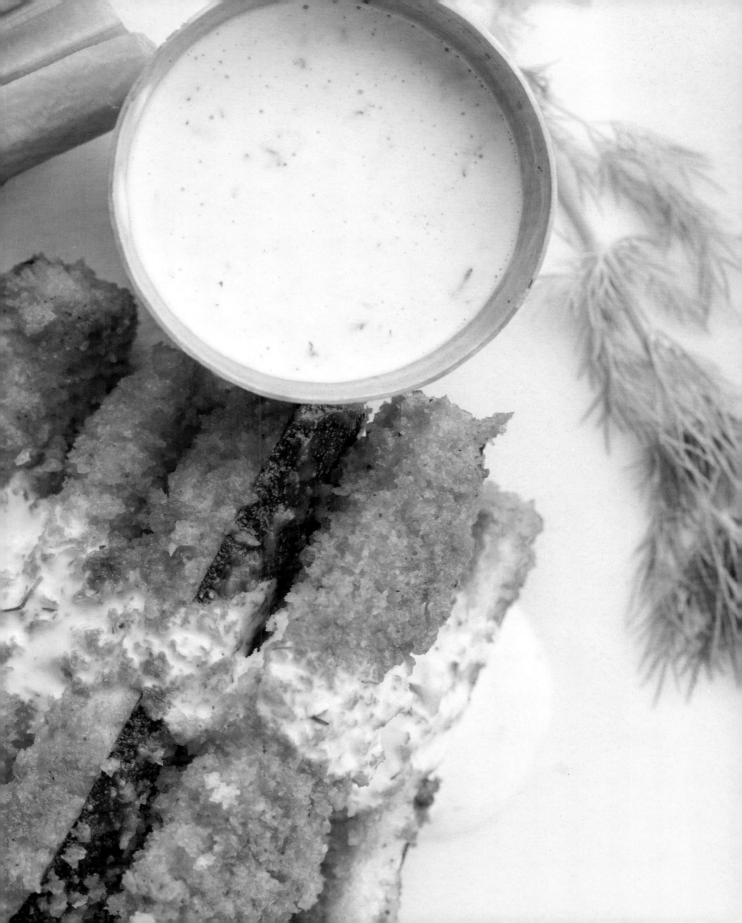

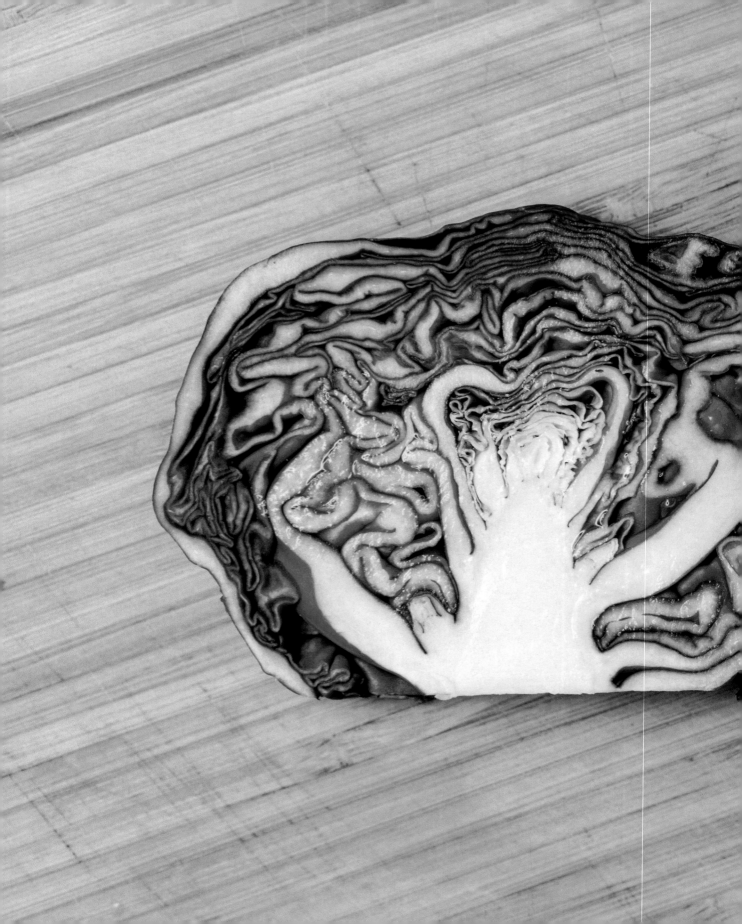

Vegetables

Butternut squash fries

SERVINGS: 6 | ◖

To ensure even cooking, cut the vegetables so all pieces are uniform in size. This recipe also works well with sweet potatoes or acorn squash.

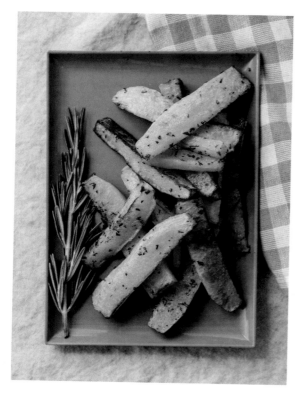

1 medium butternut squash
1 tablespoon chopped fresh thyme
1 tablespoon chopped fresh rosemary
1 tablespoon olive oil
½ teaspoon salt

Preheat oven to 425 F. Lightly coat a baking sheet with nonstick cooking spray. Peel the skin from butternut squash. Cut the squash into even sticks, about ½-inch wide and 3 inches long.

In a medium bowl, combine the squash, thyme, rosemary, olive oil and salt. Mix until the squash is evenly coated.

Spread the squash onto the baking sheet, place in the oven and roast 10 minutes. Remove baking sheet and shake to loosen the squash. Place the sheet back in the oven and continue to roast another 5-10 minutes until golden brown.

SHOPPING LIST: Butternut squash, fresh thyme, fresh rosemary

CHECK FOR: Olive oil, salt, cooking spray

NUTRITIONAL ANALYSIS PER SERVING (½ CUP): 50 calories, 2.5 g fat, 1 g protein, 8 g carbohydrates, 2 g fiber, 160 mg sodium

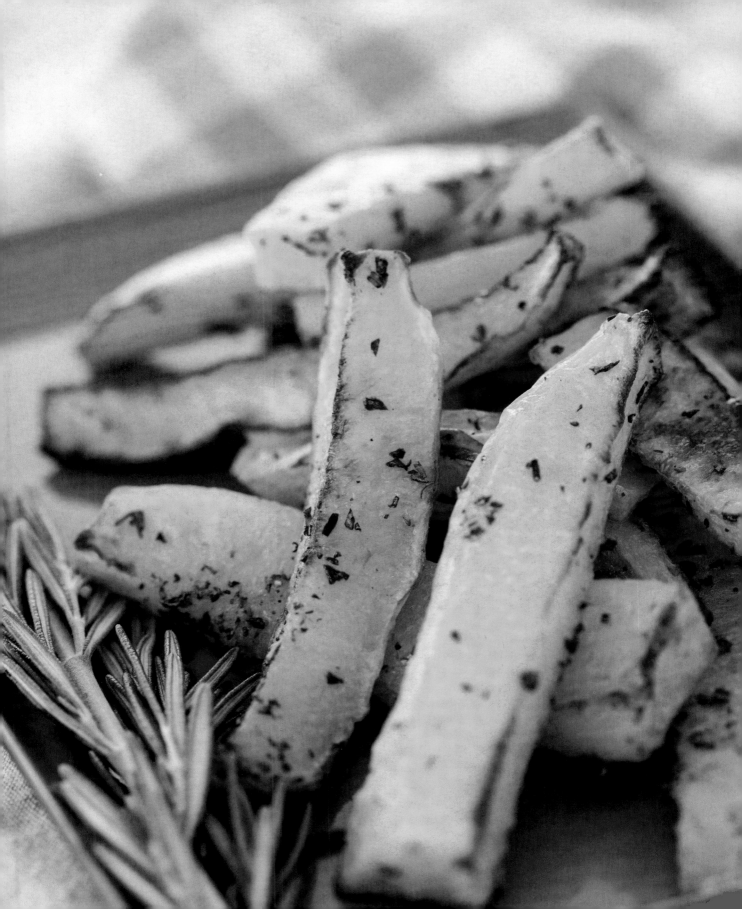

Balsamic-glazed Brussels sprouts

SERVINGS: 6 |

Blanching the Brussels sprouts before roasting them allows them to roast evenly and not burn in the oven. You can make your own balsamic glaze by slowly reducing 1 cup of balsamic vinegar with a tablespoon of sugar. Place the mixture on simmer until it's reduced by half, with about ½ cup left. This must be done slowly to create a flavorful glaze.

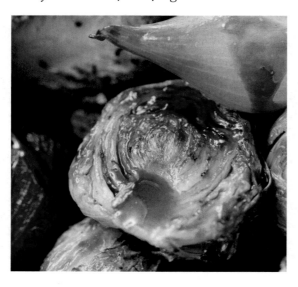

SHOPPING LIST: Brussels sprouts, red onions, balsamic glaze

CHECK FOR: Olive oil, kosher salt, pepper, cooking spray

NUTRITIONAL ANALYSIS PER SERVING (½ CUP): 60 calories, 2.5 g fat, 2 g protein, 8 g carbohydrates, 2 g fiber, 95 mg sodium

3 cups cleaned and halved Brussels sprouts
1 cup roughly chopped red onion
2 tablespoons balsamic glaze
1 tablespoon olive oil
½ teaspoon kosher salt
¼ teaspoon ground black pepper

Preheat oven to 425 F. Lightly spray a baking sheet with nonstick cooking spray. Fill a medium pot with water and bring to a boil.

Place a steamer basket over the boiling water, add the Brussels sprouts and steam approximately 3-5 minutes, depending on size of sprouts. Remove the steamer basket and drain off excess water from Brussels sprouts.

In a large bowl, mix steamed Brussels sprouts, red onion, olive oil, salt and pepper. Toss well to evenly season the Brussels sprouts and onions.

Roast 15-20 minutes, or until the vegetables are golden brown in spots (caramelized) and tender.

Drizzle the balsamic glaze over the roasted Brussels sprouts and onions and serve.

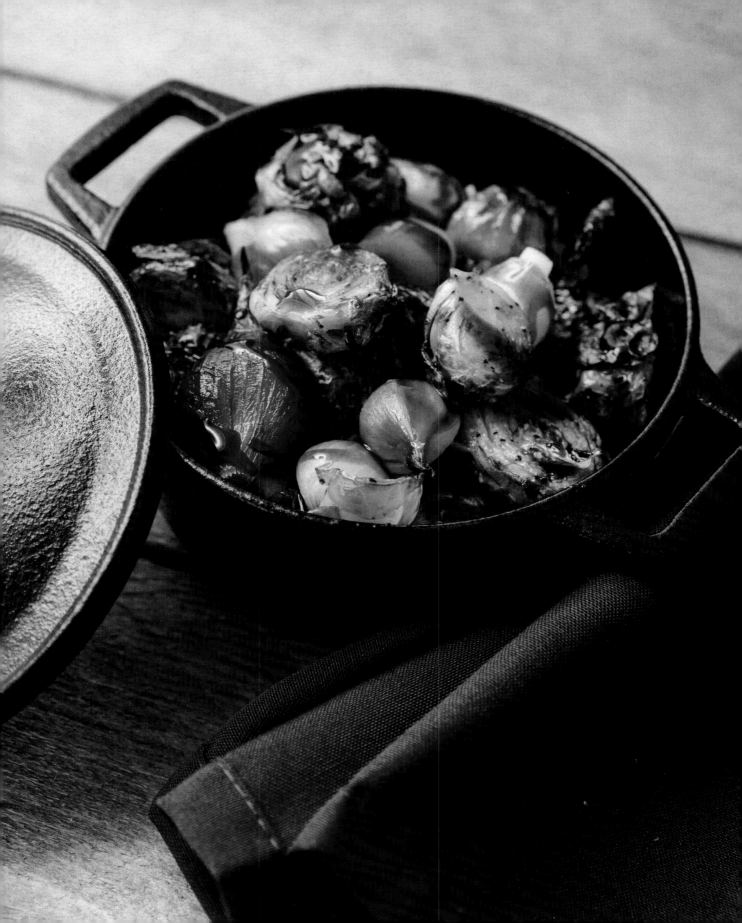

Parmesan-crusted cauliflower

SERVINGS: 6 |

This roasting technique also works well with broccoli, carrots or asparagus. Try it with your favorite vegetable for some variety.

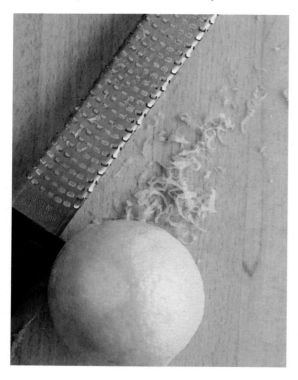

½ cup panko breadcrumbs
¼ cup finely grated fresh Parmesan cheese
  (use fresh for the best flavor)
2 tablespoons olive or canola oil
1 teaspoon fresh lemon zest
1 teaspoon finely chopped fresh basil
  or ½ teaspoon dried basil
¼ teaspoon paprika
3 cups cauliflower, chopped into 1-inch florets

Preheat oven to 375 F. Lightly coat an 8x8-inch baking dish with cooking spray. Fill a medium pot with water and bring to a boil.

In a small bowl, add the panko, cheese, oil, lemon zest, basil and paprika. Use your hands to evenly combine the mixture.

Cook the cauliflower in boiling water for 3 minutes; drain. Place the cauliflower in the baking dish and sprinkle the breadcrumb mixture evenly over the top.

Bake approximately 15 minutes or until crust is lightly brown.

SHOPPING LIST: Panko, Parmesan cheese, lemon, fresh basil (or dried), cauliflower

CHECK FOR: Olive or canola oil, paprika, cooking spray

NUTRITIONAL ANALYSIS PER SERVING (½ CUP): 100 calories, 6 g fat, 1.5 g saturated fat, 3 g protein, 10 g carbohydrates, 1 g fiber, 90 mg sodium

Honey sage carrots

If you don't have honey on hand, brown sugar is a good substitute. You can also use this recipe with butternut or acorn squash.

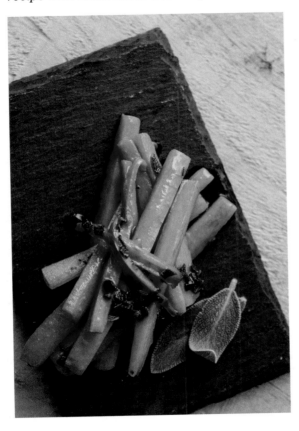

3 large carrots (approximately 2 cups), peeled and cut into sticks or half circles
1 teaspoon olive oil
1 tablespoon honey
2 tablespoons finely chopped fresh sage
¼ teaspoon kosher salt
Pinch ground black pepper or white pepper

Bring a medium pot of water to a boil while preparing the carrots. Place carrots in the boiling water and cook until tender; drain.

Preheat a medium sauté pan to medium heat or use the same pot you boiled the carrots in. Once warm, add the olive oil and carrots. Cook for about 1 minute then add the honey, sage, salt and pepper. Serve warm.

SHOPPING LIST: Carrots, honey, fresh sage

CHECK FOR: Olive oil, kosher salt, pepper

NUTRITIONAL ANALYSIS PER SERVING (½ CUP): 50 calories, 1.5 g fat, 1 g protein, 10 g carbohydrates, 2 g fiber, 160 mg sodium

Thyme-roasted beets

An alternative way to prepare this recipe is to peel and cut the beets first, coat with the oil and seasonings, and roast on a baking sheet covered with foil for approximately 20-25 minutes.

2 medium red or golden beets
1 tablespoon olive oil
1 teaspoon chopped fresh thyme
¼ teaspoon salt
¼ teaspoon ground black pepper

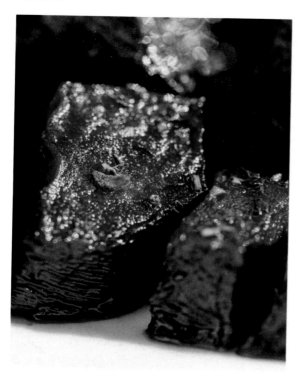

Preheat oven to 400 F. Wash and trim the beets. Wrap each in aluminum foil and bake for 40 minutes. Set aside to cool slightly.

Peel the beets and cut into medium-sized chunks. In a medium bowl, combine beets, oil, thyme, salt and pepper. Place the beets on a baking sheet and roast in the oven an additional 5-10 minutes, until hot.

SHOPPING LIST: Red or golden beets, fresh thyme

CHECK FOR: Olive oil, salt, pepper

NUTRITIONAL ANALYSIS PER SERVING (⅓ CUP): 40 calories, 2.5 g fat, 1 g protein, 4 g carbohydrates, 1 g fiber, 190 mg sodium

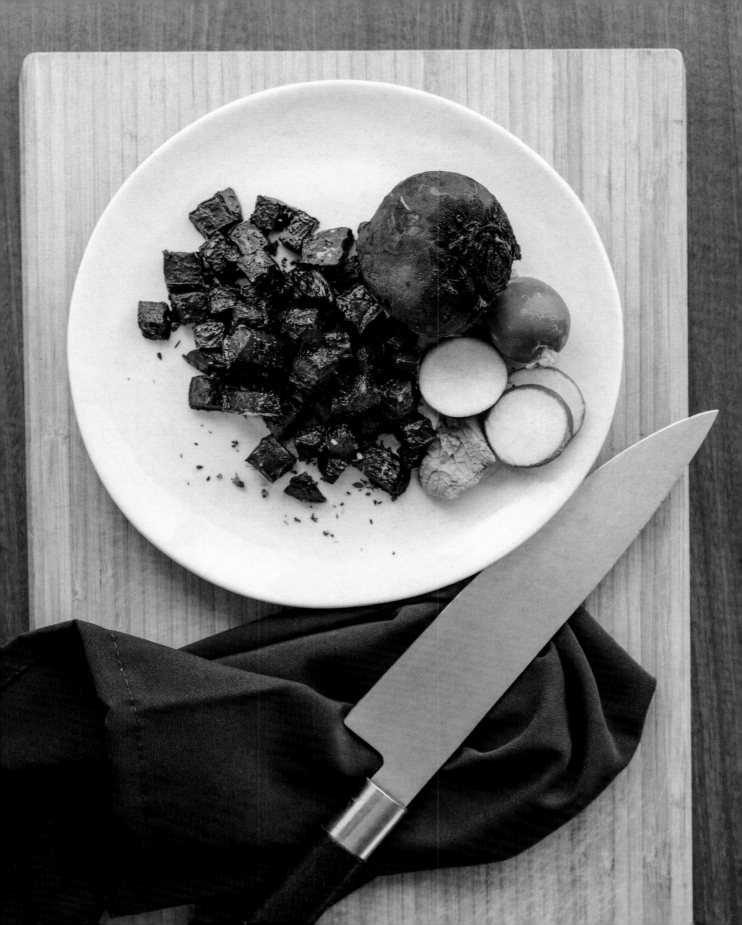

Sautéed green beans with almonds

SERVINGS: 6 |

This classic green bean recipe also works well with snow peas or sugar snap peas. If you're looking for some variety, julienned carrot sticks are a great addition to this dish.

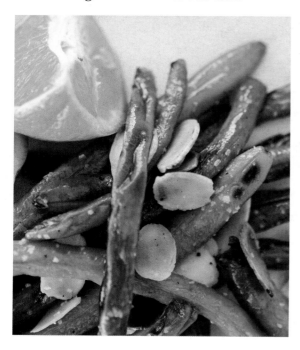

1 ½ pounds fresh green beans, cleaned and trimmed
2 teaspoons olive oil
¼ cup sliced almonds
¼ teaspoon kosher salt
¼ teaspoon ground black pepper
¼ teaspoon garlic powder

Heat a medium to large sauté pan to medium heat; add oil. Sauté green beans for approximately 5 minutes until the beans are slightly blistered. Approximately 3 minutes after adding the green beans to the pan, add the sliced almonds and sauté.

Taste a bean to see if it's done to your liking. If the beans need more time to finish cooking, add ¼ cup water.

Add the seasonings and mix well.

SHOPPING LIST: Fresh green beans, sliced almonds

CHECK FOR: Olive oil, kosher salt, pepper, garlic powder

NUTRITIONAL ANALYSIS PER SERVING (1 CUP): 80 calories, 3.5 g fat, 3 g protein, 10 g carbohydrates, 4 g fiber, 80 mg sodium

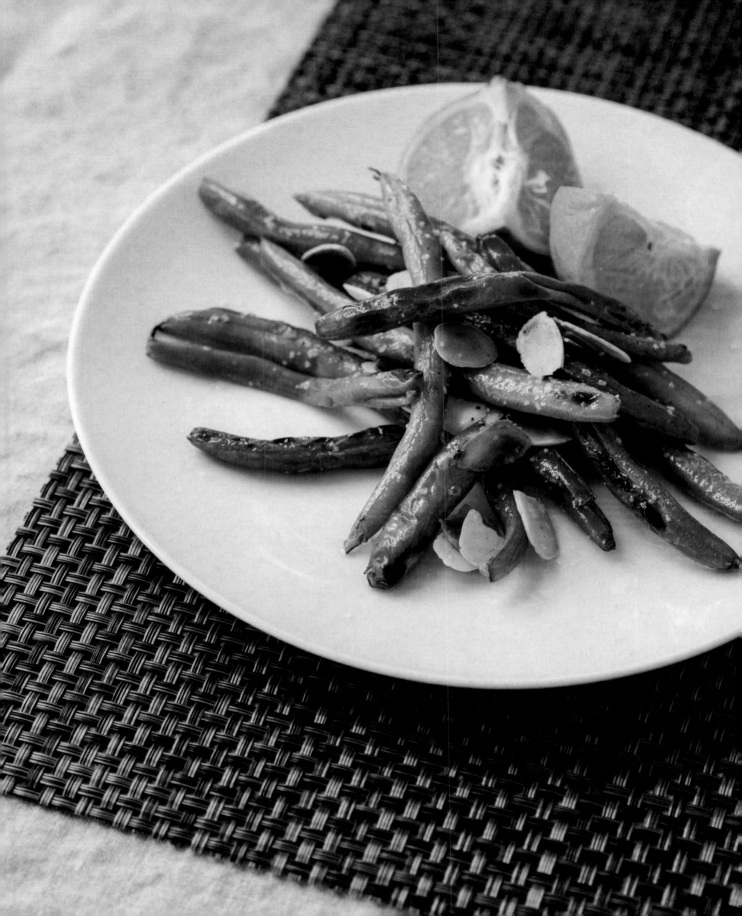

Vegetable stir-fry

You can add other vegetables, such as bean sprouts, water chestnuts, sugar snap peas or snow peas, to this dish. If you're looking for some protein, add grilled chicken breast, sautéed shrimp or tofu.

SHOPPING LIST: Fresh garlic, fresh ginger, green onion, cashews, broccoli, red bell pepper, green bell pepper, button mushrooms, onion, carrot, sesame oil, rice wine

CHECK FOR: Soy sauce

NUTRITIONAL ANALYSIS PER SERVING (1 CUP): 240 calories, 10 g fat, 1.5 g saturated fat, 16 g protein, 26 g carbohydrates, 8 g fiber, 360 mg sodium

4 cloves minced fresh garlic
2 teaspoons minced fresh ginger
1 green onion, chopped
2 tablespoons cashews
1 crown broccoli, cut into florets
1 red bell pepper, sliced
1 green bell pepper, sliced
20 button mushrooms
1 medium onion, sliced
1 large carrot, peeled and cut into half circles
1 tablespoon sesame oil
1 tablespoon reduced-sodium soy sauce
1 tablespoon cooking rice wine (mirin)

Prepare the ingredients. Heat a medium nonstick skillet to medium heat. Add the sesame oil. When the skillet is hot, add onions, peppers and ginger. Sauté 2-3 minutes.

Add the garlic, mushrooms and green onion. Once the vegetables are tender, add the broccoli and carrots. Place a lid over the skillet and steam the vegetables an additional 2-3 minutes.

Mix in soy sauce, rice wine and cashews and serve.

Herb-stuffed tomatoes

SERVINGS: 6 |

This recipe will work equally well with most types of medium to large tomatoes. Keep in mind if using a larger tomato that the servings and nutritional value per serving will change. You can make this recipe with fewer calories and less fat by omitting the ricotta cheese.

6 Roma tomatoes, washed
½ cup low-fat ricotta cheese
½ cup shredded Parmesan cheese
½ cup plain panko breadcrumbs
1 teaspoon garlic powder
½ teaspoon kosher salt
¼ cup chopped fresh basil
2 tablespoons chopped fresh oregano

Preheat oven to 400 F. Cut the tomatoes in half lengthwise and scoop out the seeds.

In a medium-sized bowl, mix the ricotta cheese, Parmesan cheese, garlic powder, salt, basil and oregano.

Scoop a heaping tablespoon of the cheese-herb mixture into each tomato half, and sprinkle with the breadcrumbs. Repeat until all tomatoes are filled.

Lightly mist the stuffed tomatoes with olive oil or nonstick cooking spray. Bake 15-20 minutes, until the breadcrumbs are lightly browned, and serve.

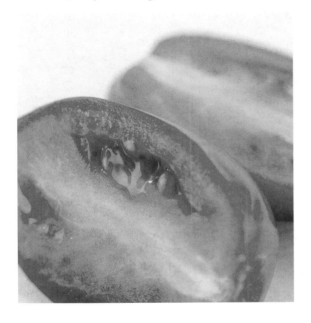

SHOPPING LIST: Roma tomatoes, low-fat ricotta cheese, Parmesan cheese, panko, fresh basil, fresh oregano

CHECK FOR: Garlic powder, kosher salt, olive oil or cooking spray

NUTRITIONAL ANALYSIS PER SERVING (2 HALVES): 100 calories, 3.5 g fat, 2 g saturated fat, 7 g protein, 11 g carbohydrates, 1 g fiber, 260 mg sodium

Grilled vegetable kebabs

SERVINGS: 6 | ●◖

Depending on the season, feel free to try different vegetables and herbs with these kebabs. For more of a fall flavor, switch out the rosemary and thyme and add fresh sage instead. Lavender or fresh dill also are great flavors to try with vegetable kebabs.

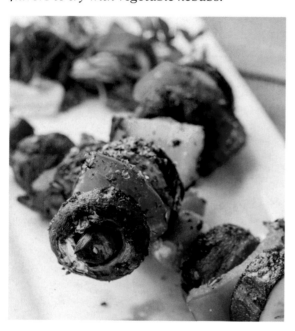

1 medium zucchini, sliced into circles
½ red bell pepper, cut into chunks
½ yellow bell pepper, cut into chunks
1 pint cherry tomatoes
10 cremini mushrooms, halved or quartered
1 red onion, cut into chunks
4 cloves garlic, minced
1 tablespoon minced fresh rosemary
1 tablespoon minced fresh thyme
2 tablespoons olive oil
½ teaspoon kosher salt
¼ teaspoon ground pepper

Soak 6 wood skewers in water for at least 30 minutes while you wash and prepare the vegetables.

Preheat a grill to medium-high heat, or use a grill pan that can accommodate the full length of the skewers.

Place all vegetables in a large bowl. Add the garlic, fresh herbs, olive oil, salt and pepper. Toss until evenly coated.

Skewer the vegetables and place on the grill (or grill pan). Turn every 2 minutes until fully cooked, totaling about 5-8 minutes. You can also partially cook the skewers on the grill, giving them great grill marks and flavor, and finish them later in a high-temperature oven.

Serve with your favorite lean protein or whole-grain entree.

SHOPPING LIST: Wood skewers, zucchini, red bell pepper, yellow bell pepper, cherry tomatoes, cremini mushrooms, red onion, garlic, fresh rosemary, fresh thyme

CHECK FOR: Olive oil, salt, pepper

NUTRITIONAL ANALYSIS PER SERVING
(1 SKEWER): 45 calories, 2.5 g fat, 1 g protein, 5 g carbohydrates, 1 g fiber, 170 mg sodium

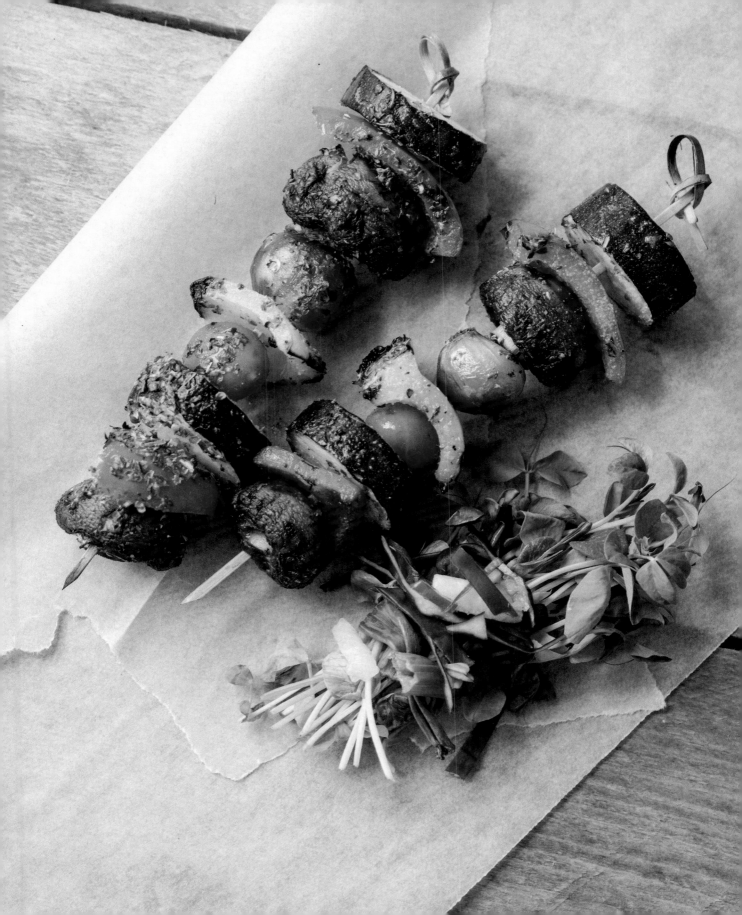

Greek roasted vegetables

The lemon, herbs and seasonings in this recipe make for a bright, summery variation on roasted vegetables. For a more substantial side of veggies, try this with a sprinkling of good-quality feta cheese on top.

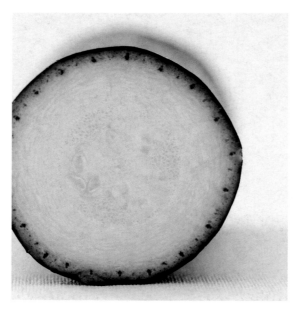

SHOPPING LIST: Zucchini, red onions, red bell peppers, yellow bell peppers or summer squash, portabella mushrooms, fresh parsley, garlic, fresh oregano

CHECK FOR: Lemon juice, olive oil, pepper, sea salt, cooking spray

NUTRITIONAL ANALYSIS PER SERVING (¾ CUP): 80 calories, 5 g fat, 0.5 g saturated fat, 2 g protein, 9 g carbohydrates, 2 g fiber, 170 mg sodium

3 medium zucchini, cut into ½-inch chunks
1 ½ red onions, cut into ½-inch chunks
1 ½ red bell peppers, cut into ½-inch chunks
1 ½ yellow bell peppers or summer squash, cut into ½-inch chunks
6 portabella mushrooms, cleaned and sliced
⅓ cup chopped fresh parsley
3 garlic cloves, minced
⅓ cup lemon juice
1 ½ teaspoons olive oil
1 ½ teaspoons chopped fresh oregano
¾ teaspoon ground black pepper
¼ teaspoon sea salt

Preheat oven to 400 F. Gather and prepare the vegetables.

In a large bowl, combine the lemon juice, olive oil, oregano, pepper and salt, and add the vegetables. Toss lightly and set aside for 10 minutes to marinate.

Lightly coat a baking sheet (15x10-inch or larger) with nonstick cooking spray. Arrange the vegetables on the pan in a single layer. Roast in oven for 20 minutes or until vegetables are crisp-tender.

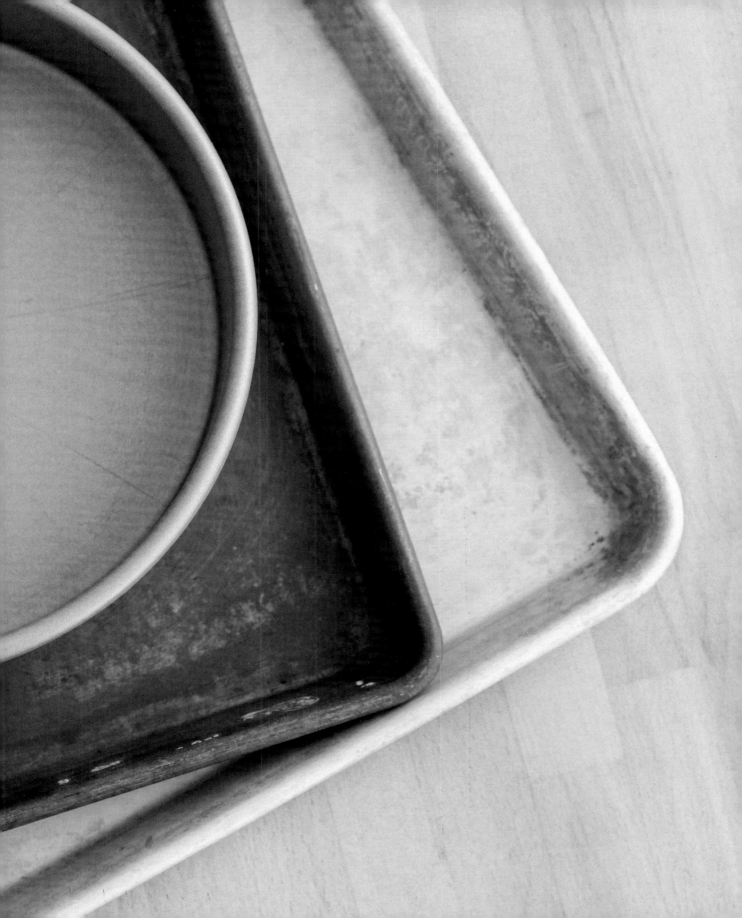

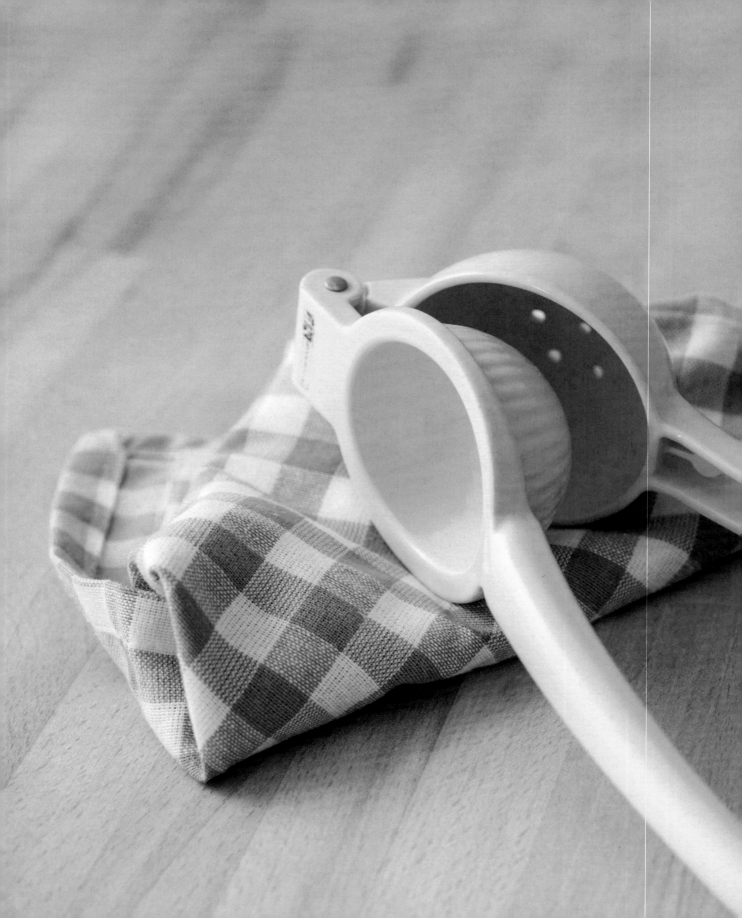

Sides

Garlic cauliflower mashed potatoes

SERVINGS: 6 |

Adding cauliflower and Greek yogurt helps reduce calories and fat while keeping the potatoes creamy. Just be sure not to overwhip the potatoes or they'll take on a paste-like texture.

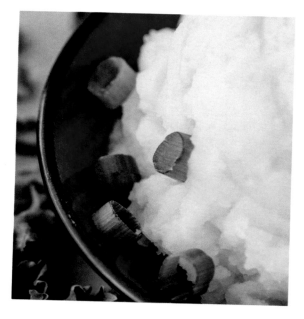

2 large russet potatoes, peeled and cut into medium-sized chunks
1 medium head cauliflower, cut into 1-inch florets
½ teaspoon finely chopped fresh thyme
1 tablespoon unsalted butter
¼ cup fat-free Greek yogurt
1 ½ teaspoons salt
½ teaspoon garlic powder
Pinch of ground black pepper

Bring water to a boil in two smaller pots or medium saucepans. Boil potatoes and cauliflower in separate pots until tender when stabbed with a fork, approximately 10 minutes. Remove from heat and drain.

Place cauliflower in a food processor and process about 2 minutes or until smooth. Place potatoes and processed cauliflower into a large mixing bowl. Using a stand mixer with a whip attachment, mix on medium speed about 1 minute. An electric hand mixer works, too. But you may need to mix the potatoes and cauliflower a little longer.

Add the thyme, butter, yogurt, salt, garlic powder and black pepper. Mix on low about 2 minutes until all ingredients are well blended, and serve.

SHOPPING LIST: Russet potatoes, cauliflower, fresh thyme, fat-free Greek yogurt

CHECK FOR: Unsalted butter, salt, garlic powder, pepper

NUTRITIONAL ANALYSIS PER SERVING (½ CUP): 90 calories, 2 g fat, 1 g saturated fat, 4 g protein, 16 g carbohydrates, 3 g fiber, 510 mg sodium

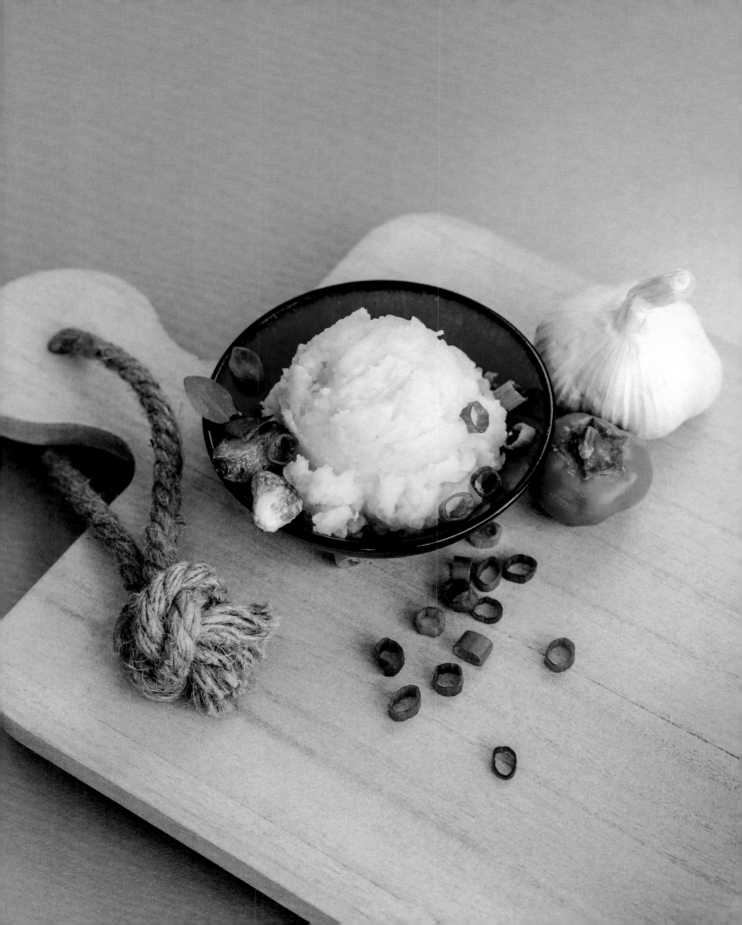

Savory mashed sweet potatoes

SERVINGS: 4 | ◗

If you have extra sweet potatoes, you can cook them with the potatoes in this recipe, and use the extra to make quinoa cakes (see page 140).

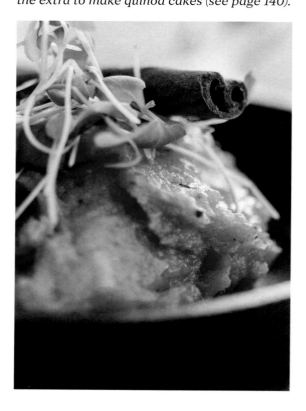

2 large sweet potatoes, peeled and cut into 1-inch chunks
1 tablespoon chopped fresh thyme
3 tablespoons fat-free plain Greek yogurt
¼ cup skim milk
½ teaspoon cinnamon
½ teaspoon salt
Pinch of nutmeg
Pinch of ground black pepper

Fill a smaller pot or medium saucepan halfway with water and bring to a boil. Prepare the sweet potatoes.

Boil the potatoes until tender when stabbed with a fork, approximately 20 minutes. Drain and set aside to cool.

In a large bowl, mash the potatoes. A stand mixer with a whip attachment works well, but you can use a potato masher. Add the thyme and remaining ingredients. Mix until well blended.

SHOPPING LIST: Sweet potatoes, fresh thyme, fat-free plain Greek yogurt

CHECK FOR: Skim milk, cinnamon, salt, nutmeg, pepper

NUTRITIONAL ANALYSIS PER SERVING (½ CUP): 70 calories, 3 g protein, 13 g carbohydrates, 2 g fiber, 270 mg sodium

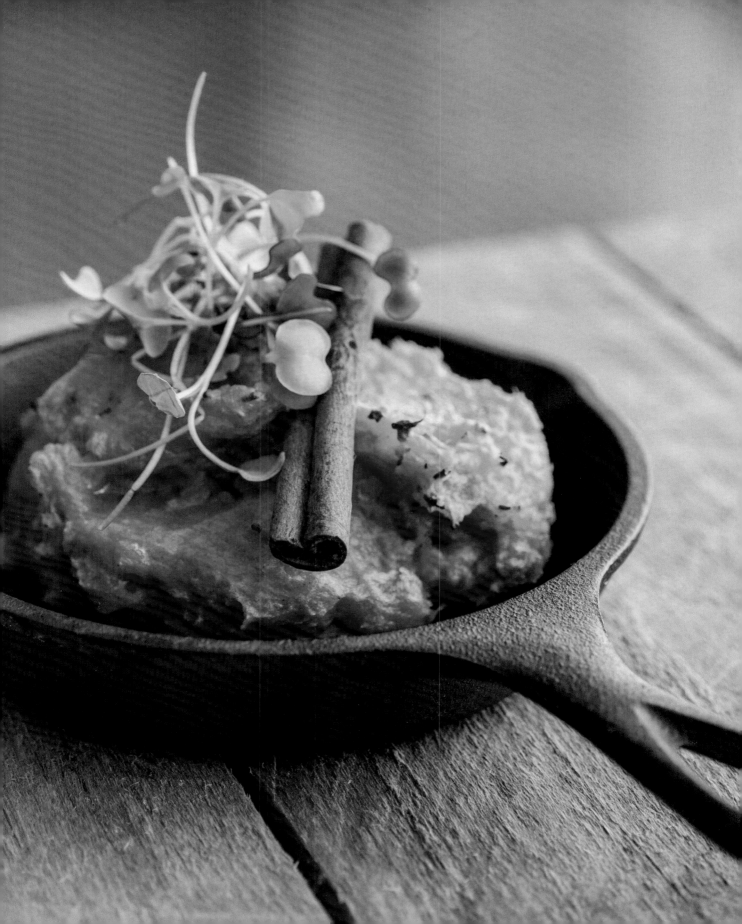

Cheesy herbed polenta

SERVINGS: 18 |

Polenta cut into circles can be grilled, baked or placed on top of casseroles. This is a generous recipe, so you may want to portion and freeze some for use later. If you'd prefer a thinner polenta, add an extra cup of water.

SHOPPING LIST: Polenta, fresh rosemary, fresh thyme, sharp 2% cheddar cheese, fresh Parmesan cheese (optional)

CHECK FOR: Salt, cooking spray

NUTRITIONAL ANALYSIS PER SERVING (½ CUP): 110 calories, 2.5 g fat, 1.5 g saturated fat, 3 g protein, 17 g carbohydrates, 1 g fiber, 170 mg sodium

6 cups water
2 cups polenta (corn grits, or coarse cornmeal)
2 tablespoons chopped fresh rosemary
2 tablespoons chopped fresh thyme
1 teaspoon salt
½ cup shredded 2% sharp cheddar cheese
Fresh Parmesan cheese (optional)

In a medium saucepan, add water and bring to a boil. As the water starts to boil, slowly pour in the polenta while whisking briskly to prevent lumps from forming in the polenta. Stir frequently.

Once the polenta absorbs the water and starts to look thick and creamy, add the salt, herbs and cheddar cheese. Remove saucepan from the heat and whisk until cheese is melted and seasonings are well blended.

Place the mixture in a pre-greased baking or cake pan or a cast iron skillet. Let the polenta cool and set up in the pan. Garnish with fresh Parmesan cheese, if desired.

Use a biscuit or round cookie cutter to cut the polenta into round shapes to form stacks. (A knife works, too.) If you have kids, use their favorite cutter to make it fun!

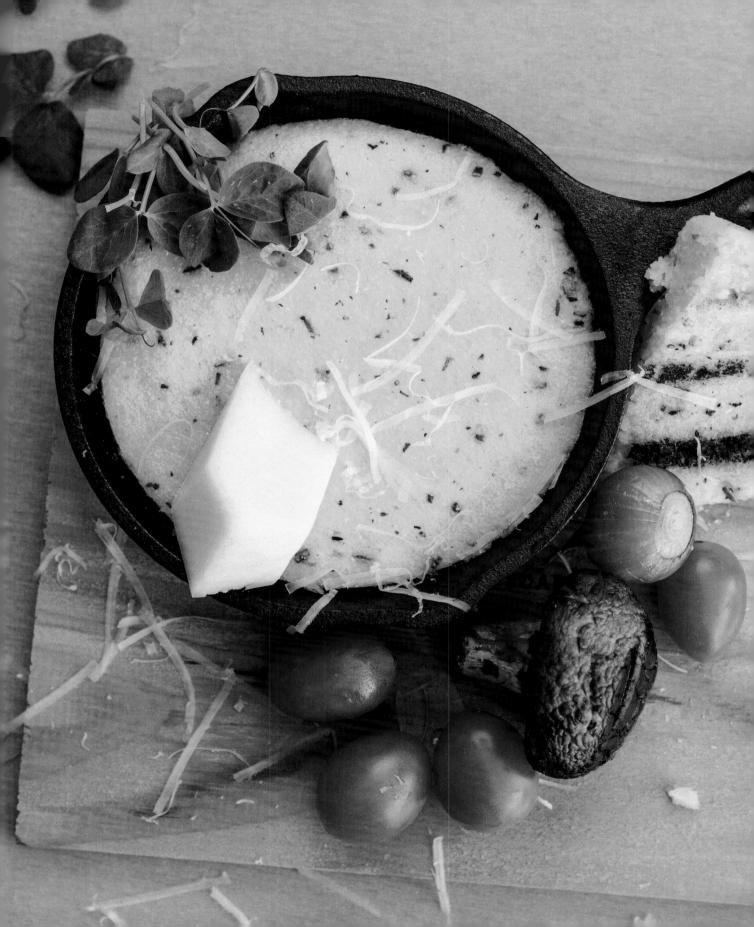

Barley risotto with vegetables

SERVINGS: 12 |

You can make this risotto with any vegetables that are in season. Try zucchini, summer squash, butternut squash, carrots, peppers and a variety of onions. Other cheeses, such as Asiago, pecorino or smoked Gouda, may be used in place of the Parmesan.

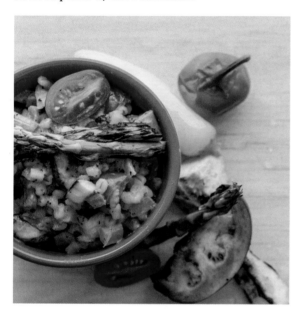

SHOPPING LIST: Barley, cremini mushrooms, asparagus, cherry tomatoes, onion, fresh thyme, low-sodium chicken stock, white wine, Parmesan cheese, half-and-half

CHECK FOR: Olive oil, kosher salt, pepper

NUTRITIONAL ANALYSIS PER SERVING (¾ CUP): 170 calories, 5 g fat, 3 g saturated fat, 8 g protein, 19 g carbohydrates, 3 g fiber, 470 mg sodium

1 cup uncooked barley
1 teaspoon olive oil
1 cup finely diced onion
1 tablespoon minced garlic
2 cups low-sodium chicken stock, divided
1 cup white wine
3 cups sliced cremini mushrooms
2 cups chopped asparagus
2 cups halved cherry tomatoes
1 ½ tablespoons chopped fresh thyme
½ cup finely grated Parmesan cheese
½ cup half-and-half
½ teaspoon kosher salt
¼ teaspoon ground black pepper

In a medium saucepan, cook the barley according to package directions.

Heat a medium sauté pan over medium-high heat. Add the olive oil and spread around the pan. Add the onion and sauté until soft. Add the barley and garlic and pour in ½ cup of the chicken stock, stirring continuously. When the liquid is absorbed, add ½ cup of white wine, stirring continuously until all the liquid is absorbed. Continue the same process, adding ½ cup of chicken stock, followed by ½ cup of wine and another ½ cup of chicken stock. (Set aside the remaining ½ cup of chicken stock.)

Add the mushrooms, asparagus, tomatoes, and thyme. When vegetables are tender, add the last ½ cup of chicken stock. When all the liquid is absorbed, add the cheese, half-and-half, salt and pepper. Reduce heat to low, stir until combined, and serve.

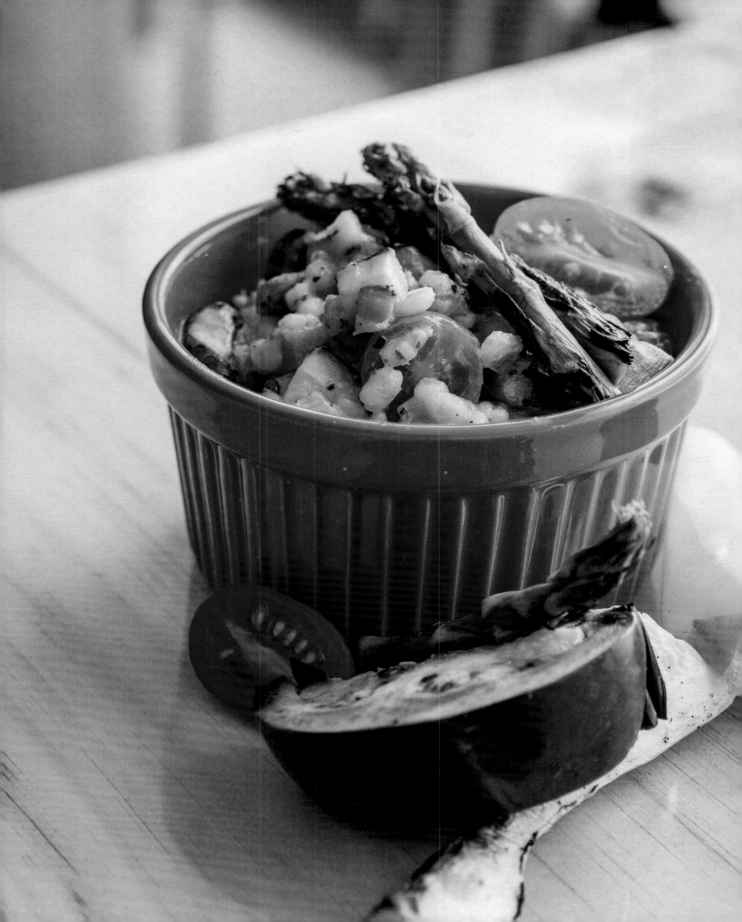

Quinoa cakes

These cakes can be prepared in advance and frozen for later use.

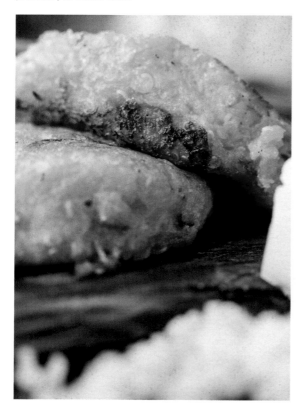

SHOPPING LIST: Quinoa, sweet potatoes, garlic, Parmesan cheese, fresh parsley

CHECK FOR: Eggs, salt, pepper, nutmeg, olive oil

NUTRITIONAL ANALYSIS PER SERVING
(1 CAKE): 220 calories, 10 g fat, 4.5 g saturated fat, 13 g protein, 21 g carbohydrates, 3 g fiber, 640 mg sodium

2 large sweet potatoes (2 cups mashed)
2 cups cooked quinoa
2 eggs
3 cloves garlic, minced
6 ounces (approximately 1 ½ cups) shredded
   Parmesan cheese
2 tablespoons finely chopped fresh parsley
1 teaspoon salt
¼ teaspoon ground black pepper
¼ teaspoon nutmeg
2 tablespoons olive oil

Preheat oven to 375 F. Spear sweet potatoes with a knife and bake until soft, approximately 45 minutes.

Cook the quinoa. Allow quinoa and sweet potatoes time to cool. Remove skin and mash the sweet potatoes.

In a large bowl, combine sweet potatoes, quinoa, eggs, garlic, Parmesan cheese, parsley, salt, pepper and nutmeg. Take amounts equaling approximately ¼ cup and form into patties.

Preheat a large sauté pan to medium-high heat and add 1 tablespoon olive oil. Cook until cakes are golden brown on both sides. Repeat process with remaining oil and quinoa mixture. Bake cakes in oven for 5 minutes to ensure they're heated through.

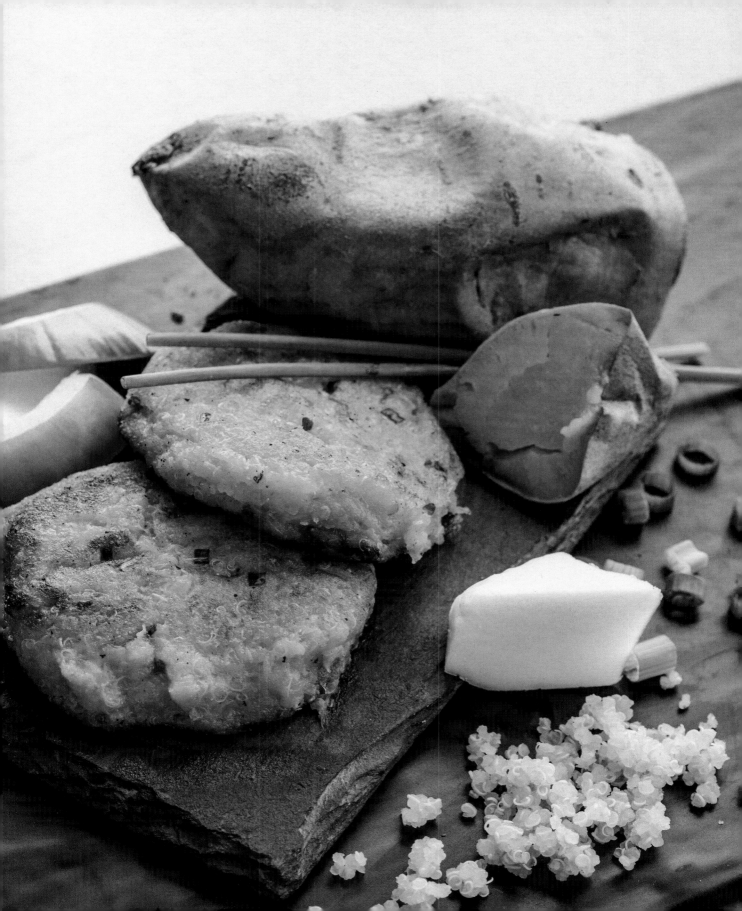

Potato cakes

SERVINGS: 8 |

Make sure to wash the potatoes well because you'll leave the potato skins on when shredding. The skins add fiber and other nutrients.

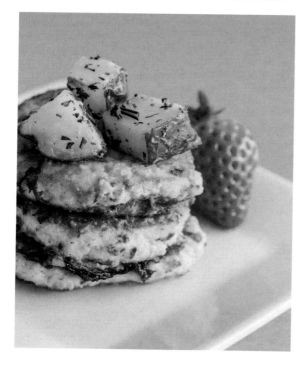

2 large baking or russet potatoes, shredded
1 ounce Parmesan or Gruyère cheese,
   shredded
1 small onion, minced, or 6 green onions,
   finely sliced
1 egg
2 tablespoons all-purpose flour
½ teaspoon salt
Ground black pepper to taste
2 teaspoons olive oil

Preheat oven to 350 F. Lightly spray a baking sheet with cooking spray.

Wash potatoes well. Use a food processor and the processor's shredding attachment to shred the potatoes. (A manual grater works, too.) Place the shredded potatoes in cold water.

In a large bowl, mix the cheese, onion, egg, flour, salt and pepper.

Drain the shredded potatoes and pat them dry. This prevents having too much moisture in your potato cakes. Add the shredded potatoes to the egg and cheese mixture and mix well. Take amounts equaling about ½ cup and form into patties.

Heat a medium or large sauté pan to medium heat and add the olive oil. Sear the cakes on each side until golden brown and place on the lightly greased baking sheet.

Bake 15-20 minutes.

SHOPPING LIST: Baking or russet potatoes, Parmesan or Gruyère cheese, onion or green onions

CHECK FOR: Eggs, flour, salt, pepper, olive oil, cooking spray

NUTRITIONAL ANALYSIS PER SERVING
(1 CAKE): 90 calories, 4 g fat, 1 g saturated fat, 4 g protein, 10 g carbohydrates, 1 g fiber, 340 mg sodium

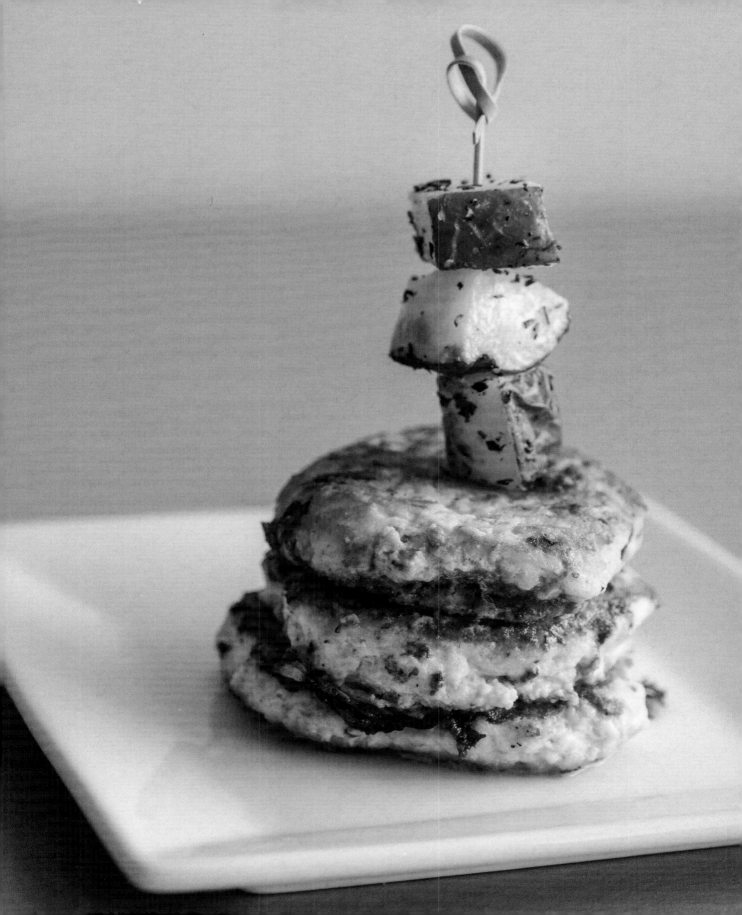

Cilantro lime rice

SERVINGS: 6 |

Depending on the size of the lime, start by squeezing half the lime and then taste the rice. Half a lime may be enough. If you accidentally add too much lime juice, add a little more butter to balance the lime's acid.

1 cup basmati brown rice
1 tablespoon unsalted butter
1 ¼ cups water
¼ teaspoon kosher salt
2 tablespoons lime juice, freshly squeezed
2 tablespoons chopped fresh cilantro

Measure the rice and set aside.

In a medium saucepan, heat the butter until melted. Add the rice and sauté approximately 2 minutes. Add the water and salt, cover and let simmer 40-50 minutes.

When the rice is done, fluff it with a fork, add the lime juice and cilantro, and serve.

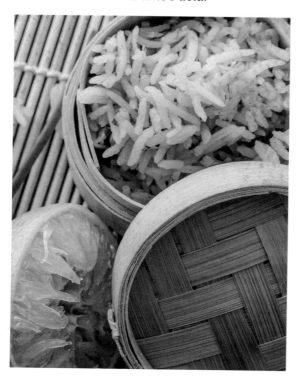

SHOPPING LIST: Basmati brown rice, lime, fresh cilantro

CHECK FOR: Unsalted butter, kosher salt

NUTRITIONAL ANALYSIS PER SERVING (½ CUP): 120 calories, 2 g fat, 2 g protein, 25 g carbohydrates, 1 g fiber, 160 mg sodium

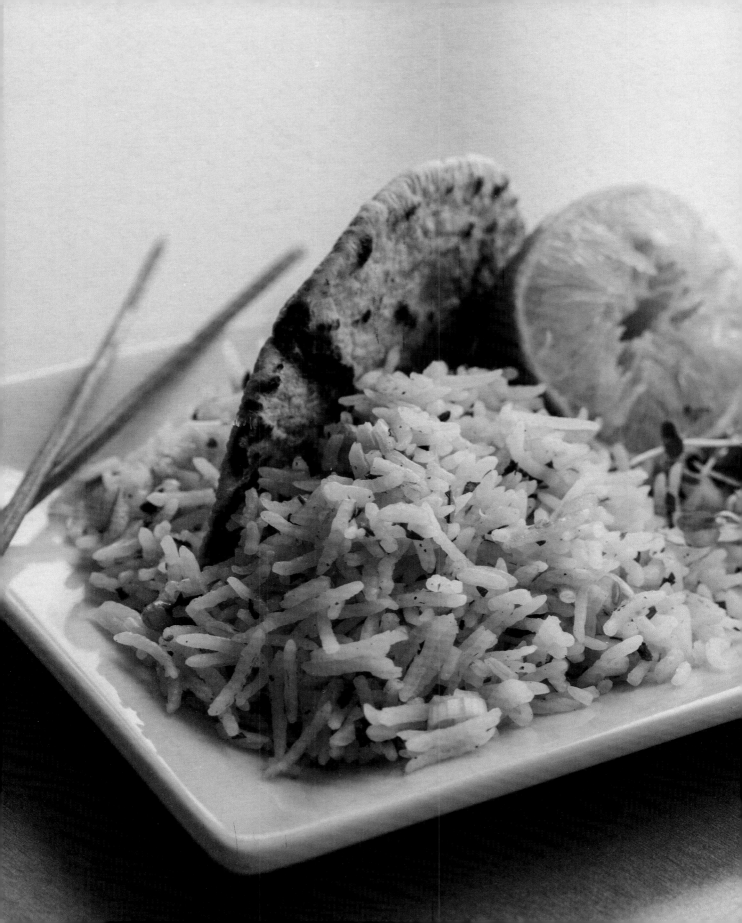

Vegetable rice pilaf

SERVINGS: 6 |

Many different vegetables, dried fruits or nuts can be added to this rice dish to change its flavor. Try dried cranberries, pecans, fresh apples, walnuts, raisins or coconut.

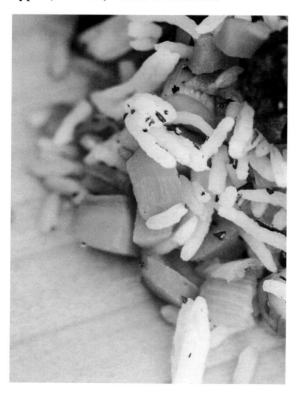

2 ¼ cups water
1 cup uncooked parboiled brown rice
1 ½ teaspoons olive oil
2 cups chopped onions
2 cups chopped carrots
2 cups chopped asparagus
1 ½ cups chopped celery
2 tablespoons finely mined fresh thyme
1 teaspoon salt

In medium saucepan, bring water and rice to a boil. Once boiling, lower heat to a simmer and cover. Cook the rice until water is completely absorbed. Spread the rice on a baking sheet to cool.

Warm a large nonstick sauté pan to medium heat. Add the oil and sauté the onions, carrots and celery.

When the onions, carrots and celery are tender, add the rice, asparagus, thyme and salt. Mix until combined and warmed through.

SHOPPING LIST: Parboiled brown rice, onions, carrots, asparagus, celery, fresh thyme

CHECK FOR: Olive oil, salt

NUTRITIONAL ANALYSIS PER SERVING (1 ¾ CUP): 160 calories, 2.5 g fat, 4 g protein, 33 g carbohydrates, 4 g fiber, 350 mg sodium

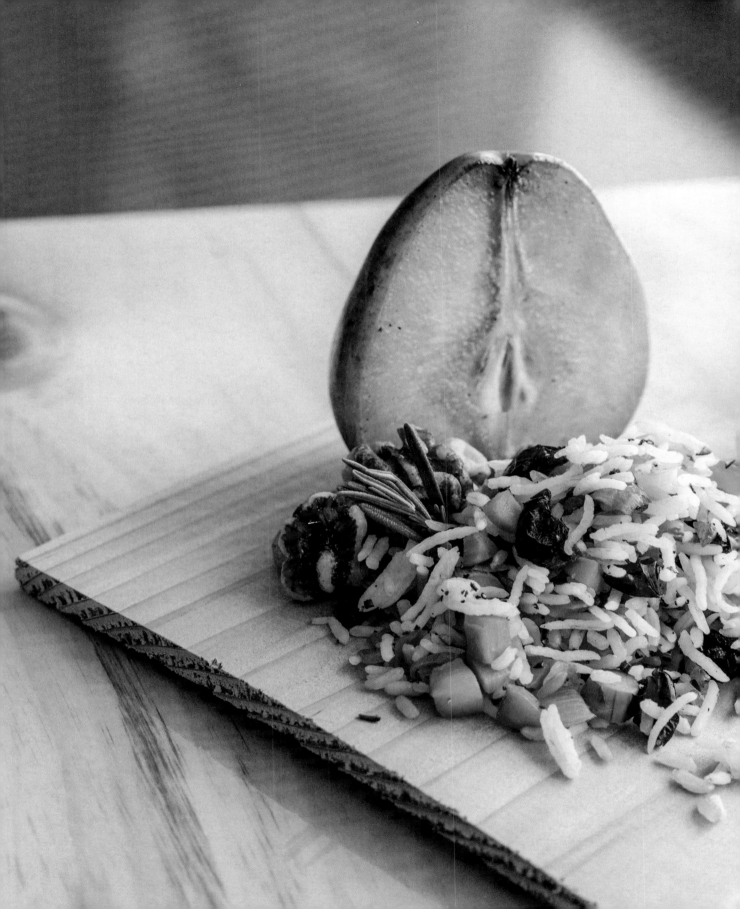

Mango cilantro slaw

Try changing up this slaw by adding different fruit, such as fresh pineapple, nectarines or peaches. In addition to tacos, enjoy this slaw with barbecue sandwiches.

⅛ cup chopped shallots
1 cup diced mango
1 bunch fresh cilantro, finely chopped
¾ cup rice vinegar
¼ cup rice wine (mirin)
2 tablespoons sugar
3 ½ cups grated cabbage, or a pre-shredded
   mix
1 ¼ cup grated carrots
¼ cup chopped red onion

Combine all ingredients in a medium bowl. Let sit and marinate 1-2 hours before serving.

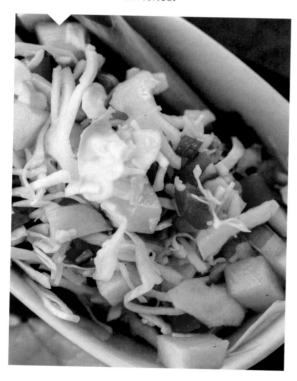

SHOPPING LIST: Shallots, mango, cilantro, rice vinegar, rice wine (mirin), cabbage, carrots, red onion

CHECK FOR: Sugar

NUTRITIONAL ANALYSIS PER SERVING (¾ CUP): 130 calories, 6 g fat, 1 g protein, 21 g carbohydrates, 2 g fiber, 95 mg sodium

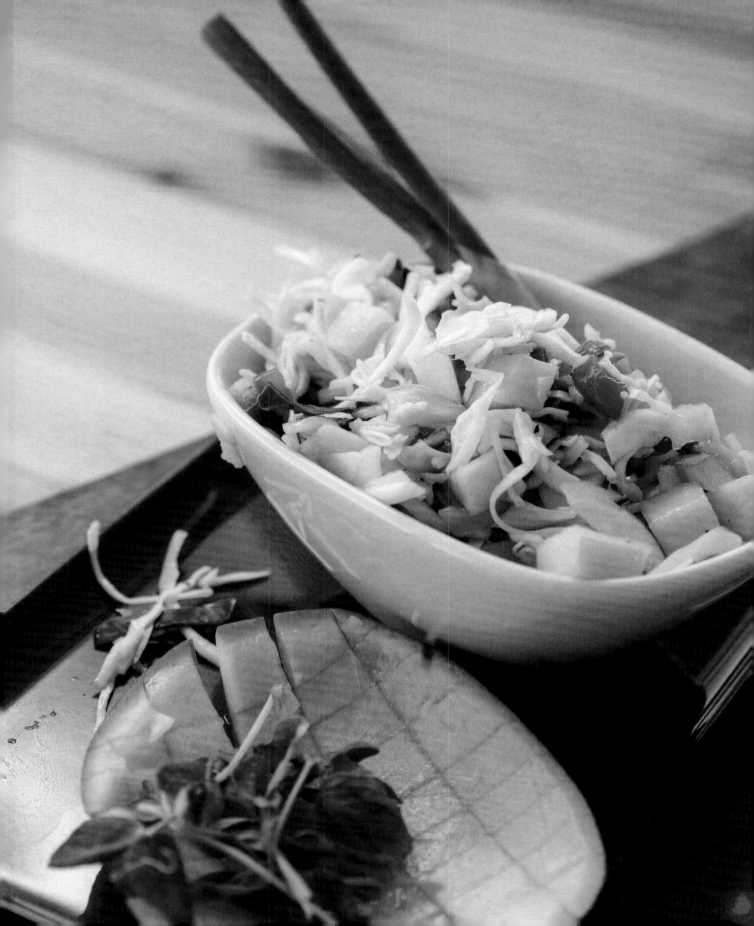

Orange jicama slaw

Jicama is a root vegetable with thick, brown skin that's native to Mexico. It has a potato- and pear-like texture and provides a slightly sweet earthy flavor. Jicama makes a great slaw.

⅛ cup chopped shallots
1 cup orange segments
¾ cup rice vinegar
¼ cup rice wine (mirin)
2 tablespoons sugar
3 ½ cups grated jicama
1 ¼ cup grated carrots
¼ cup sliced red onion

Combine all ingredients in a medium bowl. Let sit and marinate 1-2 hours before serving.

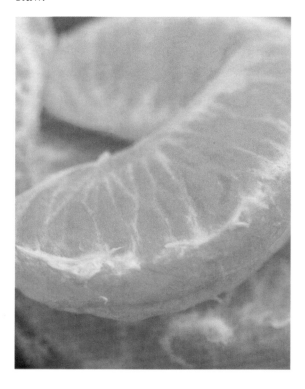

SHOPPING LIST: Shallots, orange, rice vinegar, rice wine (mirin), jicama, carrots, red onion

CHECK FOR: Sugar

NUTRITIONAL ANALYSIS PER SERVING (¾ CUP): 60 calories, 1 g protein, 15 g carbohydrates, 4 g fiber, 80 mg sodium

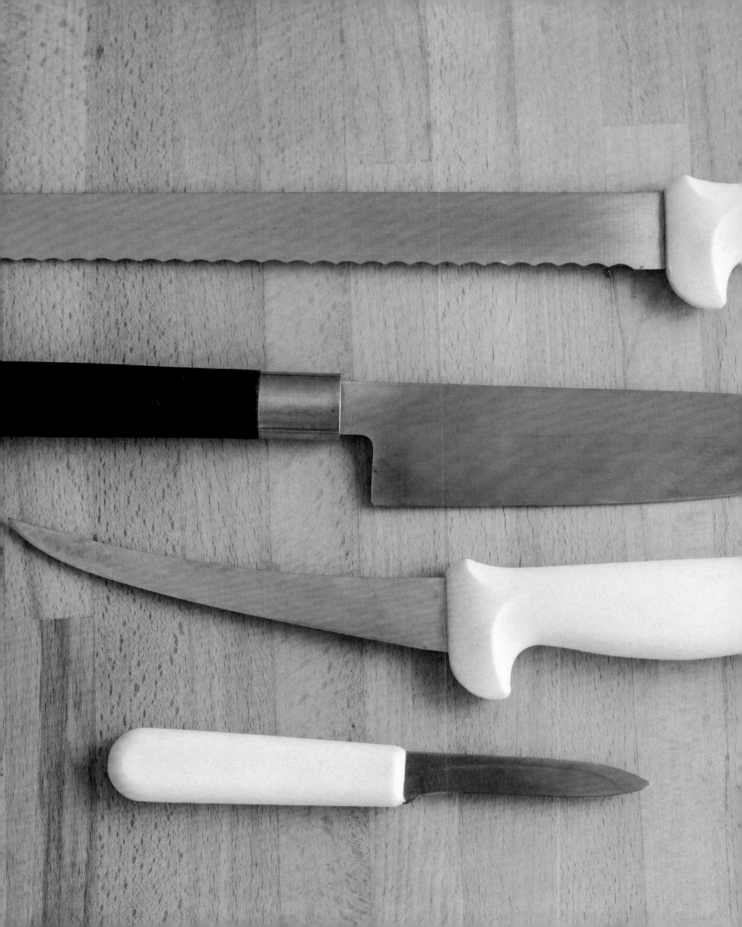

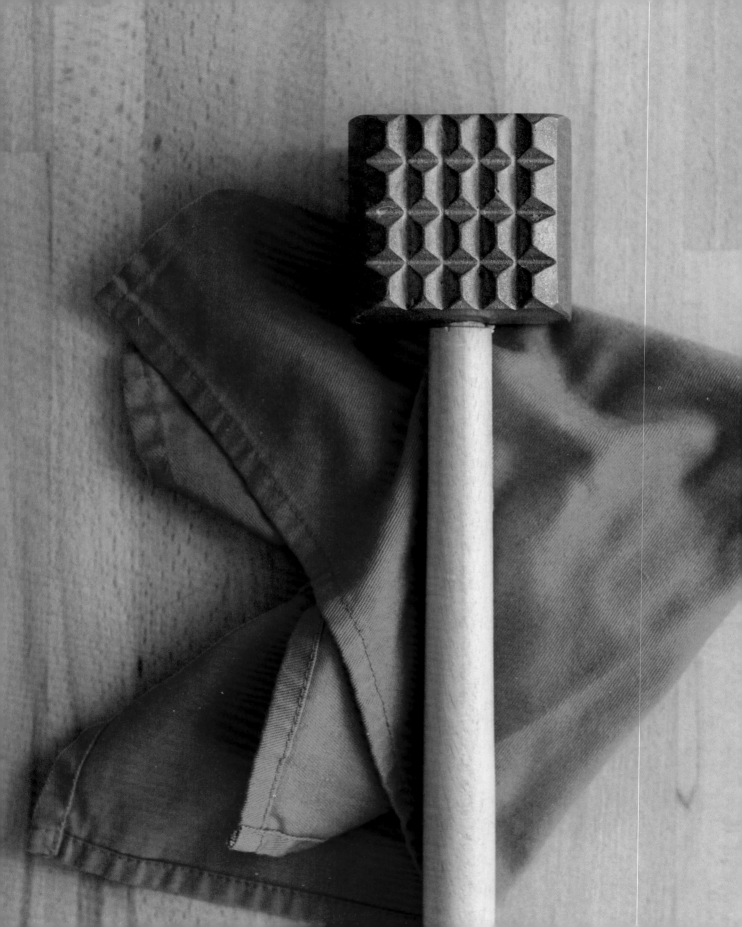

Entrees with meat or fish

Lemon chicken

SERVINGS: 4 |

The chicken stock in this dish should thicken in the pan. If a thicker sauce is desired, slowly add a small amount of cornstarch slurry. To make a slurry, combine ¼ cup cold water and ¼ cup cornstarch in a small bowl. Mix well before adding to stock.

1 teaspoon finely chopped fresh rosemary
4 (4-ounce) boneless, skinless chicken breasts
¼ cup whole-wheat flour
1 teaspoon ground black pepper
¼ teaspoon kosher salt
1 tablespoon canola oil
¼ cup lemon juice
1 cup unsalted chicken stock

Using a mallet, pound out chicken breasts to ¼-inch thickness.

In a medium bowl, combine the rosemary, flour, pepper and salt. Dredge the chicken breasts in the flour mixture and place on a baking sheet.

Heat a large nonstick sauté pan to medium heat. Add the oil and spread it around in pan. Once the oil is hot, add the chicken and cook for 4 minutes on each side. After flipping the chicken, add the lemon juice and cook another 2 minutes to let the juice evaporate or absorb into the chicken. Add the chicken stock and let it reduce and thicken a few more minutes.

Plate the chicken, and pour the remaining sauce over the top. Garnish with lemon zest or roasted tomato, if desired.

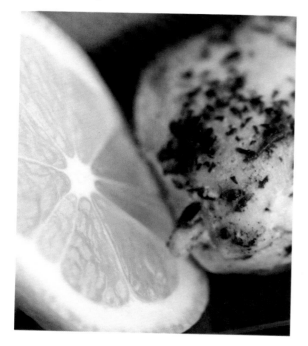

SHOPPING LIST: Fresh rosemary, boneless skinless chicken breasts, whole-wheat flour, lemon juice, unsalted chicken stock

CHECK FOR: Pepper, kosher salt, canola oil

NUTRITIONAL ANALYSIS PER SERVING (1 BREAST): 190 calories, 6 g fat, 1 g saturated fat, 27 g protein, 2 g carbohydrates, 320 mg sodium

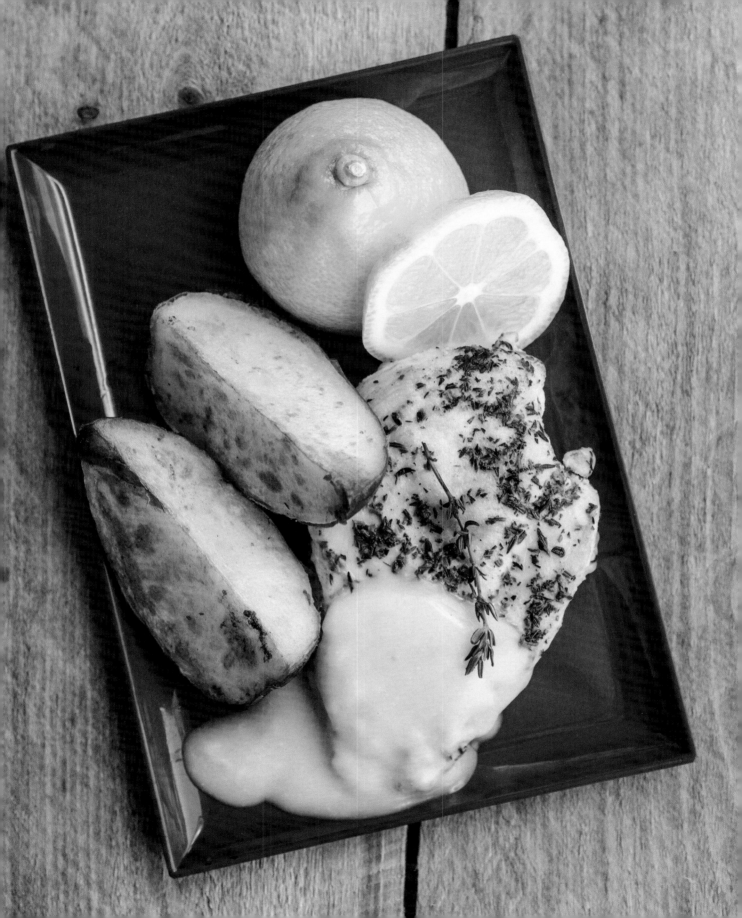

Chicken Parmesan

SERVINGS: 4 |

For an even coating on the chicken, place the panko, Parmesan cheese and seasonings in a food processor and pulse together. This ensures the panko and grated cheese are even in size and consistency.

SHOPPING LIST: Boneless skinless chicken breasts, panko, Parmesan cheese, marinara sauce, part-skim mozzarella cheese

CHECK FOR: Eggs, basil, oregano, garlic powder, onion powder, cooking spray

NUTRITIONAL ANALYSIS PER SERVING (1 BREAST): 390 calories, 11 g fat, 5 g saturated fat, 42 g protein, 27 g carbohydrates, 4 g fiber, 700 mg sodium

4 (4-ounce) boneless, skinless chicken breasts
2 egg whites
1 cup panko breadcrumbs
½ cup finely grated Parmesan cheese
2 teaspoons dried basil
2 teaspoons dried oregano
1 teaspoon garlic powder
1 teaspoon onion powder
2 cups marinara sauce
½ cup shredded part-skim mozzarella cheese

Preheat oven to 375 F. Using a mallet, pound each chicken breast to ¼-inch thickness; set aside.

Place the egg whites in a medium bowl. In another medium bowl, combine the panko, Parmesan cheese, basil, oregano, garlic powder and onion powder.

Coat a baking sheet with cooking spray. Dip each chicken breast into the egg whites, then dredge in the breading mixture until evenly coated. Lay chicken fillets on the baking sheet. Bake 15-20 minutes or until chicken is golden brown and reaches an internal temperature of 165 F.

Top the chicken with marinara sauce and mozzarella cheese and serve.

Santa Fe lime fajitas

SERVINGS: 8 |

The citrusy marinade for these fajitas also pairs well with chicken, fish, pork or even tofu, especially when used with quesadillas, burritos and tacos.

SHOPPING LIST: Beef tenderloin, lime juice, chicken or vegetable stock, fresh cilantro, garlic, sweet onion, green bell peppers, 6-inch flour tortillas

CHECK FOR: Pepper, sea salt or kosher salt

NUTRITIONAL ANALYSIS PER SERVING (1 FAJITA): 320 calories, 20 g fat, 4 g saturated fat, 20 g protein, 3 g fiber, 700 mg sodium

1 pound beef tenderloin, trimmed extra lean, cut into strips
1 cup lime juice, fresh or concentrate
4 cups chicken or vegetable stock
½ cup chopped fresh cilantro
1 tablespoon minced garlic
1 tablespoon cracked black pepper
¼ teaspoon sea salt or kosher salt
1 sweet onion, julienned
2 green bell peppers, sliced
8 (6-inch) corn tortillas, warmed

Mix the lime juice, chicken or vegetable stock, cilantro, garlic, pepper, and salt together in a deep bowl. Place the beef tenderloin strips in the mixture and marinate for at least 20 minutes.

Preheat cast iron skillet or grill. Placed the marinated strips on the hot grill or skillet for 4-8 minutes, depending on the preferred doneness.

Preheat a nonstick sauté pan over medium to medium-high heat. Add the peppers and onions and sauté about 3 minutes, or until just softened.

Assemble approximately 2 ounces of beef with a few slices of onion and peppers in each tortilla and serve.

Blackened fish tacos

If mahi-mahi isn't available, you can make these tacos with any other whitefish, such as cod or halibut, or even shrimp.

4 (3-ounce) mahi-mahi fillets, or bigger fillets
   cut into 3-ounce servings
1 tablespoon blackening spice (see below)
4 flour tortillas, warmed
1 cup roasted red pepper pineapple salsa
   (see below)
½ avocado, chopped
¼ cup feta crumbled cheese

BLACKENING SPICE | 16 SERVINGS
2 teaspoons paprika
1 teaspoon ground dried thyme
2 teaspoons onion powder
2 teaspoons garlic powder
1 tablespoon sugar
2 teaspoons salt
1 teaspoon ground black pepper
½ teaspoon cayenne pepper
1 teaspoon dried oregano
½ teaspoon ground cumin

ROASTED RED PEPPER PINEAPPLE SALSA | 6 SERVINGS
1 cup cored and cubed fresh pineapple
½ cup roasted and chopped red bell pepper
1 jalapeno, seeded and diced
¼ cup chopped fresh cilantro
¼ cup chopped red onion
¼ teaspoon salt
2 teaspoons honey

BLACKENING SPICE
Mix dry ingredients together in small bowl. Store remaining spice in an air-tight container.

ROASTED RED PEPPER PINEAPPLE SALSA
Combine all ingredients in a medium bowl. Cover and refrigerate until ready to serve.

TACOS
Preheat the grill. Rub mahi-mahi with blackening spices for at least 4-5 minutes. Lightly coat with cooking spray on each side of fish fillets.

Grill fish for 3-4 minutes a side, depending on size of fillet, until you reach an internal temperature of 140 F.

To assemble tacos, place a warm tortilla on a plate. Top with 1 ½ ounces fish, ¼ cup roasted red pepper pineapple salsa, ¼ of the chopped avocado, and 1 tablespoon feta cheese.

SHOPPING LIST: Mahi-mahi, flour tortillas, avocado, feta cheese, fresh pineapple, red bell pepper, jalapeno, fresh cilantro, red onion

CHECK FOR: Paprika, thyme, onion powder, garlic powder, sugar, salt, pepper, cayenne pepper, oregano, cumin, honey, cooking spray

NUTRITIONAL ANALYSIS PER SERVING (1 TACO): 280 calories, 7 g fat, 1.5 g saturated fat, 21 g protein, 34 g carbohydrates, 460 mg sodium

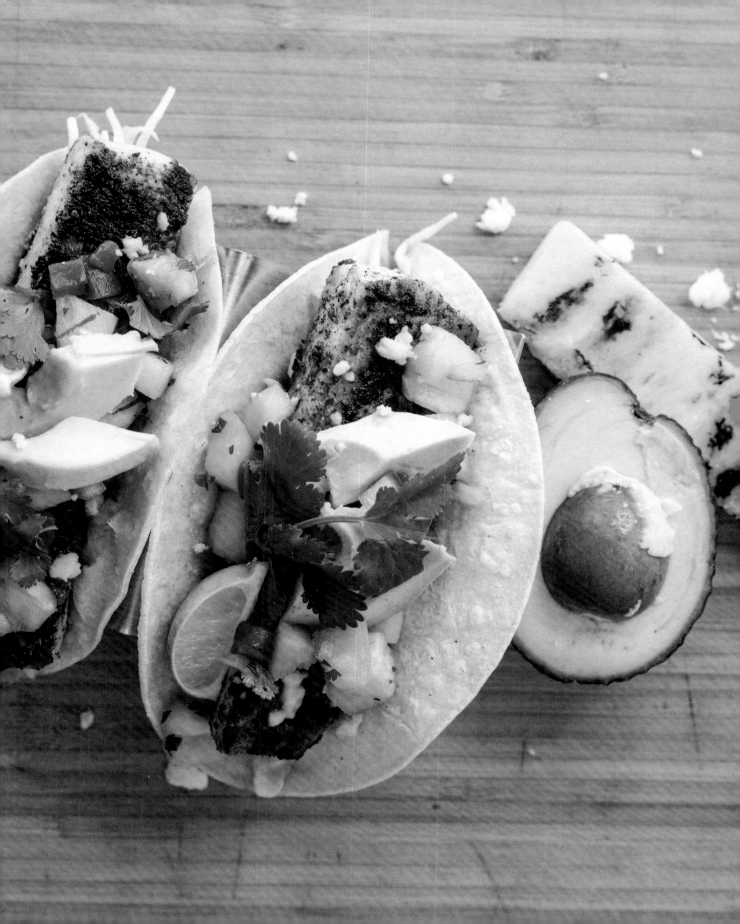

Crabcakes

Searing each crabcake in a sauté pan will provide a crisp crust. Sear cakes on both sides for about 1-2 minutes, then place on baking sheet and finish by baking in the oven.

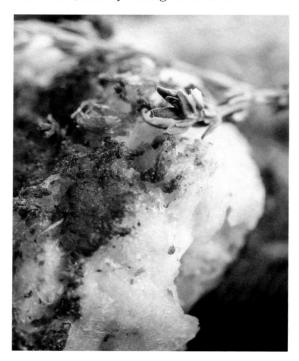

1 can (16 ounces) crabmeat
¼ cup Egg Beaters or 2 egg whites
3 tablespoons reduced-fat mayonnaise
1 tablespoon lemon juice
2 teaspoons Dijon mustard
2 teaspoons fresh dill
½ teaspoon Old Bay seasoning
½ cup panko or whole-wheat breadcrumbs

Preheat oven to 350 F. In a large bowl, combine all ingredients; mix well.

Using a scale, divide mixture into 4-ounce cakes. Set cakes aside.

Place the breadcrumbs in a small bowl. Toss each crabcake in the breadcrumbs one at a time to coat. Once coated, place cakes on a baking sheet.

Bake crabcakes for 20 minutes until cakes are browned on top.

SHOPPING LIST: Crabmeat, Egg Beaters or egg whites, lemon juice, fresh dill, Old Bay seasoning, panko or whole-wheat breadcrumbs

CHECK FOR: Reduced-fat mayonnaise, Dijon mustard

NUTRITIONAL ANALYSIS PER SERVING
(1 CAKE): 100 calories, 1 g fat, 12 g protein, 9 g carbohydrates, 520 mg sodium

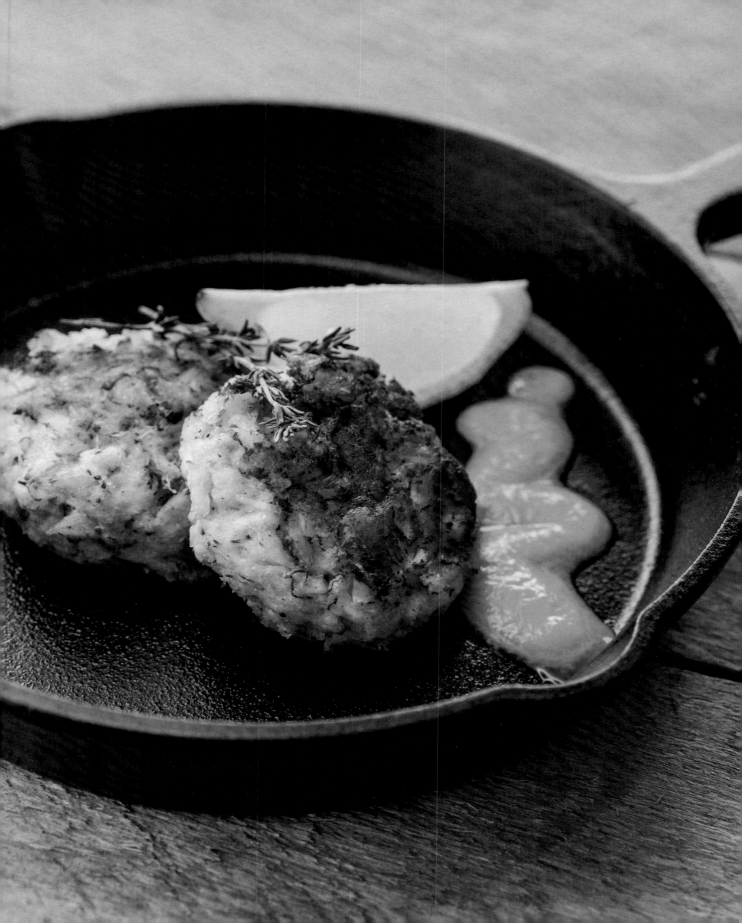

Dijon Parmesan salmon

Cod, trout or other whitefish can be substituted for the salmon. Keep a close watch on the cooking time; fish can become dry if overcooked. When cooking fillets with a small amount of oil, you may need to lower the heat. Anticipate longer cooking time if the heat needs to be lowered.

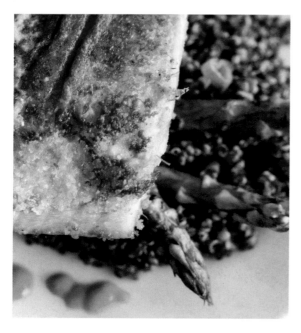

¼ cup Dijon mustard
2 tablespoons reduced-fat mayonnaise
¼ cup grated Parmesan cheese
¼ cup panko breadcrumbs
4 (4-ounce) salmon fillets
¼ teaspoon salt
¼ teaspoon ground black pepper
2 teaspoons olive oil

Preheat oven to 375 F. In a small bowl, combine the mustard and mayonnaise. In another small bowl, combine the cheese and breadcrumbs.

Coat the top of each salmon fillet with 1 ½ tablespoons of the mustard mixture and 2 tablespoons of the breadcrumb mixture. Sprinkle each fillet with salt and pepper.

Heat a large nonstick pan to medium-high heat; add oil. Cook fillets for 1 minute or until golden brown. If the pan is ovenproof, place it in the oven to finish cooking, or place fillets on a baking sheet crusted side up. Bake for approximately 6 minutes or until salmon flakes with a fork.

SHOPPING LIST: Parmesan cheese, panko, salmon fillets

CHECK FOR: Dijon mustard, reduced-fat mayonnaise, salt, pepper, olive oil

NUTRITIONAL ANALYSIS PER SERVING (4 OUNCES): 240 calories, 9 g fat, 2.5 g saturated fat, 28 g protein, 6 g carbohydrates, 600 mg sodium

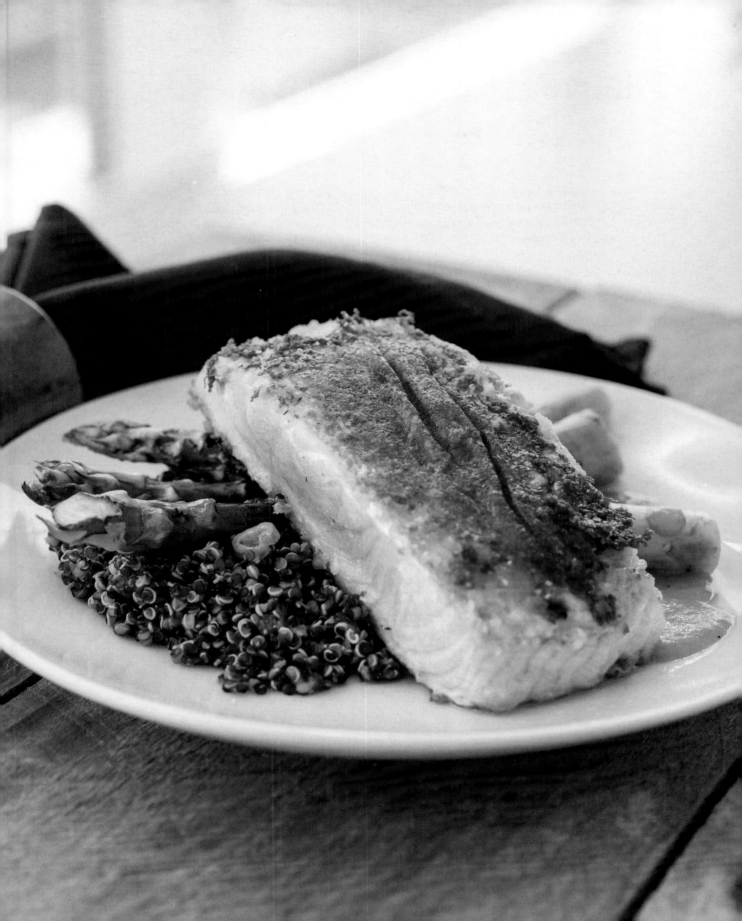

Macadamia-crusted walleye

When seasoning fish or meat, test a small amount of the seasoning mixture before applying it to the fish or meat so you can adjust the seasoning to your liking.

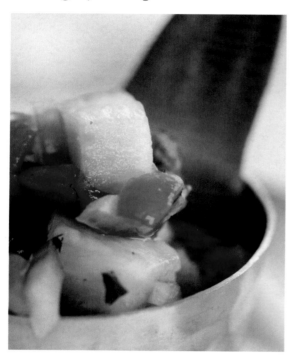

SHOPPING LIST: Fresh parsley, macadamia nuts, panko, walleye fillets

CHECK FOR: Kosher salt, garlic powder, onion powder, pepper, olive oil

NUTRITIONAL ANALYSIS PER SERVING (4 OUNCES): 290 calories, 16 g fat, 2.5 g saturated fat, 24 g protein, 13 g carbohydrates, 1 g fiber, 330 mg sodium

1 tablespoon chopped parsley
6 tablespoons macadamia nuts
6 tablespoons panko breadcrumbs
2 (4-ounce) walleye fillets
¼ teaspoon kosher salt
¼ teaspoon garlic powder
¼ teaspoon onion powder
Pinch ground black pepper
1 teaspoon olive oil

In a food processor, combine nuts and breadcrumbs; pulse until mixture reaches an even consistency.

In a small bowl, combine the parsley, nut and breadcrumb mixture, salt, garlic powder, onion powder, and pepper. Coat the top of each fillet (not the skin side) with approximately half of the seasoning.

Heat a large sauté pan to medium-high heat; add oil. Sear the seasoned side of the fillet for about 1 minute, then carefully flip over and lower the heat to medium. Cover and let cook for approximately 2-3 minutes. Walleye should flake when done. Use a meat thermometer to check for an internal temperature of 145 F.

Roasted red pepper pineapple salsa makes a great accompaniment (page 158).

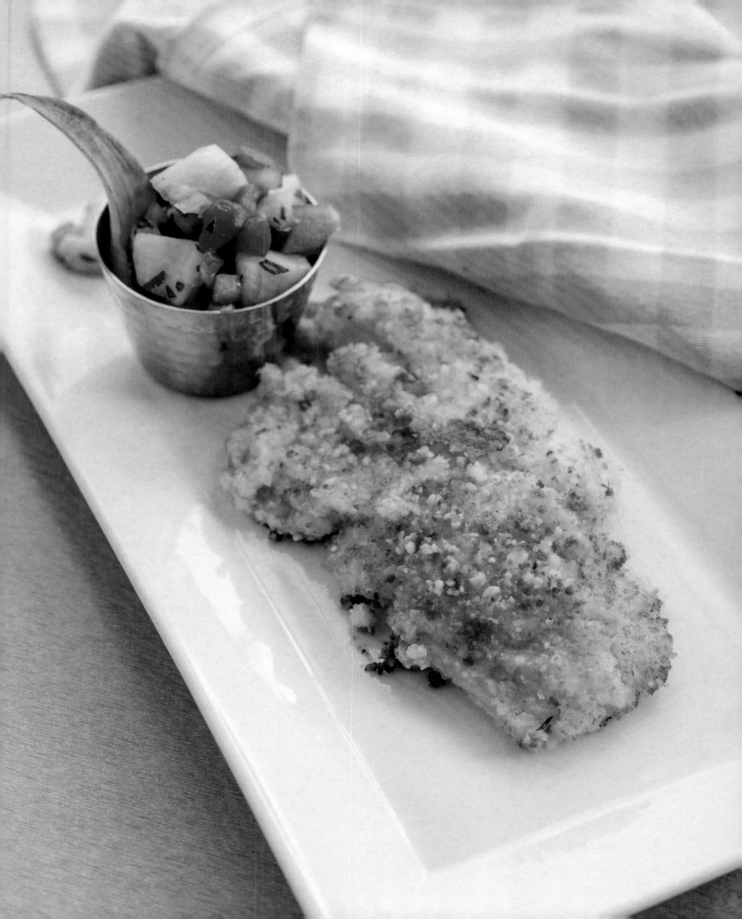

Tuscan shrimp with sun-dried tomatoes and spinach

SERVINGS: 4 |

This is a fairly quick-cooking recipe, so be sure to have all ingredients ready to add to the pan. If you'd prefer a thicker, creamier sauce, you can add 2 ounces of low-fat cream cheese to thicken the sauce a bit more. If you're not a fan of shrimp, this recipe can also be made with thin slices of beef or chicken breast.

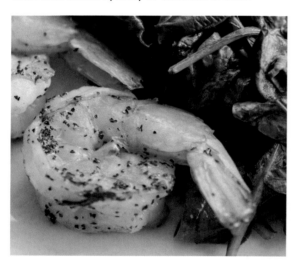

SHOPPING LIST: Shrimp, spinach, sun-dried tomatoes, chardonnay or other dry white wine, fresh basil, heavy cream, unsalted chicken stock, Parmesan cheese, pasta

CHECK FOR: Olive oil, garlic

NUTRITIONAL ANALYSIS PER SERVING (¼ RECIPE): 310 calories, 12 g fat, 5 g saturated fat, 25 g protein, 16 g carbohydrates, 4 g fiber, 890 mg sodium

1 tablespoon olive oil
1 pound shrimp, peeled and deveined
8 cups spinach, stems removed
1 cup sun-dried tomatoes
1 tablespoon minced garlic
1 cup chardonnay or other dry white wine
½ cup chopped fresh basil
¼ cup heavy cream
1 cup unsalted chicken stock
¼ cup shredded Parmesan cheese
4 ounces favorite pasta

Prepare pasta in small pot. Heat a large nonstick pan to medium-high heat. When the pan is hot, add the olive oil. Add the spinach, sun-dried tomatoes and garlic, stirring frequently.

Once the spinach is nicely wilted, move all ingredients to one side of the pan. Add the shrimp to the other side.

Let shrimp sear about 30 seconds before turning them over. Then stir the spinach mixture and shrimp together.

Add the wine and reduce the heat to medium or low. Once the wine has reduced by about half, add the remaining ingredients and simmer approximately 2 minutes. Serve over the pasta.

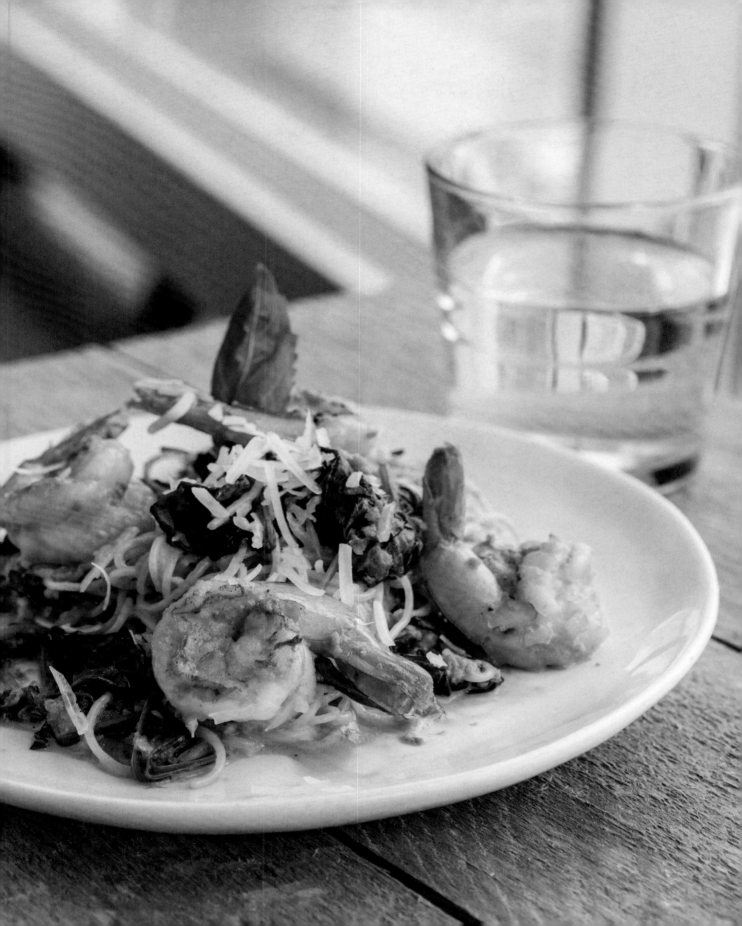

Maple balsamic pork tenderloin

SERVINGS: 4 |

This pork is juicy and flavorful on its own. For a delicious variation, serve it with the apple cider compote on page 244.

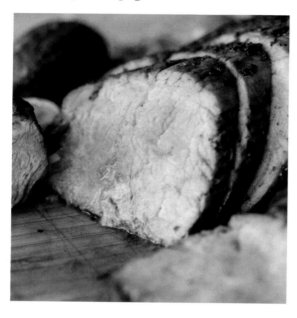

SHOPPING LIST: Pork tenderloin, balsamic vinegar, maple syrup, fresh rosemary, fresh thyme, shallot

CHECK FOR: Sea salt, white pepper, garlic, parchment paper or cooking spray

NUTRITIONAL ANALYSIS PER SERVING (APPROX. 3 OUNCES)*: 210 calories, 3.5 g fat, 1.5 g saturated fat, 22 g protein, 23 g carbohydrates, 580 mg sodium

Includes a third of the marinade that's likely absorbed by the meat.

1 pound plain pork tenderloin, cleaned and trimmed
1 teaspoon sea salt
¼ teaspoon ground white pepper

MARINADE
½ cup balsamic vinegar
½ cup maple syrup
1 tablespoon chopped fresh rosemary
1 tablespoon chopped fresh thyme
1 tablespoon minced garlic
1 finely chopped shallot

In a small bowl, mix together the marinade ingredients. Combine the pork tenderloin with the marinade in a baking dish or airtight bag and let marinate at least 1 hour.

Remove tenderloin from the marinade. To make the sauce, place the marinade in a saucepan at medium heat until it reduces and thickens slightly.

Preheat oven to 350 F. Place parchment paper on a baking sheet, or spray the baking sheet with cooking spray. Place the tenderloin on the baking sheet and season with salt and pepper.

Bake 20 minutes or until the meat reaches an internal temperature of 135 F. This temperature will cook the pork to medium-rare. If you prefer medium-well, cook to 155 F.

Slice tenderloin at a slight angle and serve with the reduced sauce.

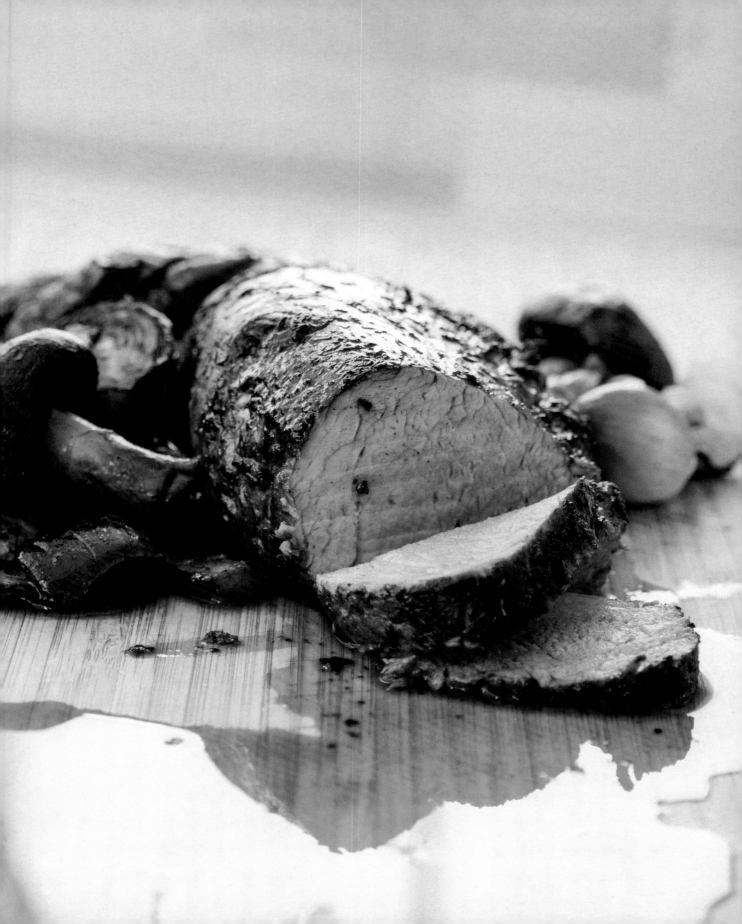

Herb-roasted pork tenderloin

SERVINGS: 4 |

Roasting the meat in convection mode will help maintain the crispy, seared crust, and cooking will go faster than in conventional mode. For a sweet and savory combination, try serving with a peach or apple compote, or another favorite sauce.

SHOPPING LIST: Fresh rosemary, fresh thyme, apple cider vinegar, pork tenderloin

CHECK FOR: Pepper, salt

NUTRITIONAL ANALYSIS PER SERVING (APPROX. 3 OUNCES): 120 calories, 3.5 g fat, 1.5 g saturated fat, 22 g protein, 1 g carbohydrates, 570 mg sodium

2 tablespoons chopped fresh rosemary
2 tablespoons chopped fresh thyme
1 cup apple cider vinegar
1 teaspoon ground black pepper
½ teaspoon salt
1 (1-pound) pork tenderloin

Preheat oven to 375 F. In a medium bowl, combine rosemary, thyme, apple cider vinegar, pepper and salt.

Trim pork tenderloin of silver skin and fat. Place in a shallow baking dish. Add the marinade so it covers the tenderloin. Let marinate at least 20 minutes.

Heat a large nonstick sauté pan to medium-high heat. Sear pork tenderloin, rotating occasionally until all sides are browned.

Place tenderloin on a baking sheet and bake 15-20 minutes or until reaching an internal temperature of 140-145 F. If a well-done center is desired, cook to 160 F. Slice at an angle and serve.

Sweet and savory meatloaf

SERVINGS: 8 |

The lean ground turkey breast adds protein with fewer calories and less fat per serving compared with using all beef. Ground chicken breast and ground pork tenderloin can be used in place of the turkey or the beef.

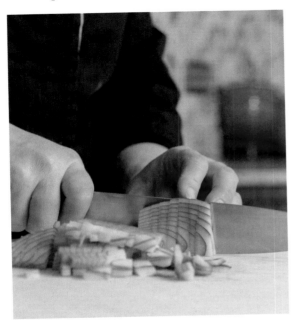

12 ounces lean ground beef (93% or 95% lean)
12 ounces ground turkey breast
¼ cup brown sugar
½ cup ketchup
1 egg
2 tablespoons egg whites
½ cup skim milk
1 teaspoon kosher salt
¼ teaspoon ground black pepper
1 cup finely diced onion
¾ cup panko breadcrumbs

Preheat oven to 350 F. Place all ingredients in a medium mixing bowl and combine so the ingredients are evenly distributed.

Spray a 9x5-inch loaf pan lightly with cooking spray. Place meatloaf mixture in the pan.

Place parchment paper over the pan, then cover that with aluminum foil. The parchment helps seal the moisture in to keep the lean meat from drying out.

Bake 35 minutes, until the center of the meatloaf reaches an internal temperature of 160 F. Gently remove from the pan and slice, or slice in the pan, and serve.

SHOPPING LIST: Lean ground beef, ground turkey breast, onion, panko

CHECK FOR: Brown sugar, ketchup, eggs, skim milk, kosher salt, pepper, cooking spray, parchment paper, aluminum foil

NUTRITIONAL ANALYSIS PER SERVING
(3 OUNCES COOKED): 210 calories,
4.5 g fat, 1.5 g saturated fat, 22 g protein,
22 g carbohydrates, 490 mg sodium

Turkey burgers

SERVINGS: 2 |

Use a thermometer to ensure you don't overcook and dry out the turkey burgers. They'll continue cooking for a few minutes after being taken off the heat, so cook them to an internal temperature of 160 F. Allow them to rest a few minutes until they reach an internal temperature of 165 F.

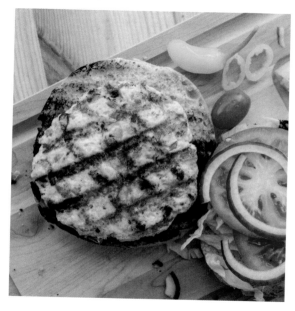

SHOPPING LIST: Ground turkey breast, onion, fresh cilantro, eggs, panko, whole-wheat buns

CHECK FOR: Garlic powder, onion powder, cumin, salt, pepper, cooking spray

NUTRITIONAL ANALYSIS PER SERVING (1 BURGER): 200 calories, 3 g fat, 0.5 g saturated fat, 30 g protein, 13 g carbohydrates, 1 g fiber, 580 mg sodium

½ pound ground turkey breast
½ cup onion
½ teaspoon garlic powder
½ teaspoon onion powder
½ teaspoon ground cumin
2 tablespoons chopped fresh cilantro
½ teaspoon salt
¼ teaspoon ground black pepper
1 egg
¼ cup panko breadcrumbs (to be used if mixture is too wet)
2 whole-wheat buns

Chop the onion in a food processor. In a medium bowl, mix the turkey breast, onion, garlic powder, onion powder, cumin, cilantro, salt, pepper and egg.

Heat a grill or medium sauté pan to medium heat. Lightly coat the grill or pan with cooking spray. Form the burger mixture into two 4-ounce patties. If the mixture is too wet, add the panko.

Place the patties on the grill or in the pan and cook approximately 5 minutes on each side or until they reach an internal temperature of 160 F. Remove the patties from the heat and let rest until reaching a temperature of 165 F.

Place the patties onto the buns and serve with your choice of condiments.

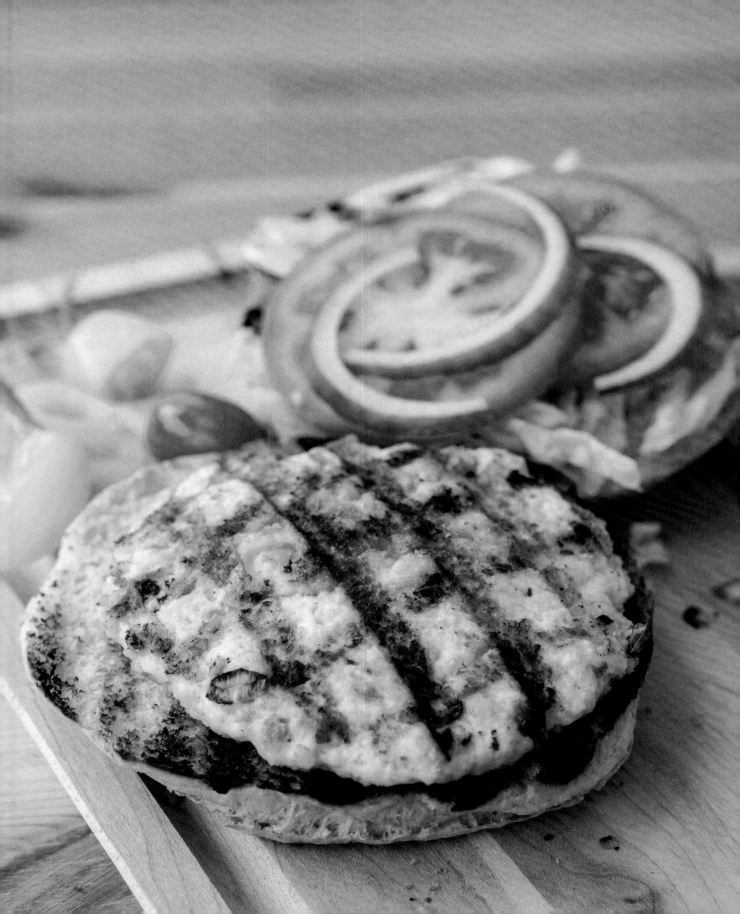

Hearty beef lasagna

SERVINGS: 12 |

This lasagna takes some time to prepare and cook, but it can be assembled a day ahead of time and refrigerated until you're ready to put it in the oven. You could also roast the vegetables a day ahead of time so assembly is faster.

3 cups broccoli florets, cut small
3 cups diced zucchini
3 cups diced yellow squash
1 tablespoon olive oil
1 ½ teaspoons garlic powder
¼ teaspoon salt
3 cups 1% cottage cheese
¾ cup shredded part-skim mozzarella cheese
½ cup shredded Parmesan cheese
12 whole-wheat lasagna noodles (sheets)
2 pounds lean ground beef
1 onion, diced
1 teaspoon garlic powder
1 teaspoon salt
1 teaspoon dried basil
½ teaspoon dried oregano
3 ½ cups marinara sauce, divided
1 teaspoon Italian seasoning
1 teaspoon garlic powder
2 tablespoons chopped fresh Italian parsley

Preheat oven to 425 F. Gather and prepare the vegetables and toss with the olive oil, garlic powder and salt. Spread on a baking sheet and roast 15 minutes. Remove and reduce oven temperature to 350 F.

In a large sauté pan at medium-high heat, add ground beef, diced onion and spices. Brown the beef, stirring occasionally. When browned, add 3 cups of the marinara sauce.

Spray a 9x13-inch baking pan with cooking spray. Spread ¼ cup marinara sauce on the bottom. Layer with 4 lasagna sheets, half the roasted vegetables, and 1 ½ cups cottage cheese. Top with half the meat sauce. Repeat with 4 lasagna sheets, veggies, cottage cheese and meat sauce and one more row of lasagna sheets. Top last layer with ¼ cup marinara sauce.

Cover with parchment paper and aluminum foil. Bake at 350 F for 1 hour and 15 minutes. Remove covering, top with mozzarella and Parmesan, and bake 5-10 minutes longer to lightly brown the cheese.

SHOPPING LIST: Broccoli, zucchini, yellow squash, cottage cheese, mozzarella cheese, Parmesan cheese, lasagna noodles, ground beef, onion, marinara sauce, fresh Italian parsley

CHECK FOR: Olive oil, garlic powder, salt, basil, oregano, Italian seasoning, cooking spray

NUTRITIONAL ANALYSIS PER SERVING (1 PIECE): 400 calories, 12 g fat, 5 g saturated fat, 41 g protein, 29 g carbohydrates, 4 g fiber, 760 mg sodium

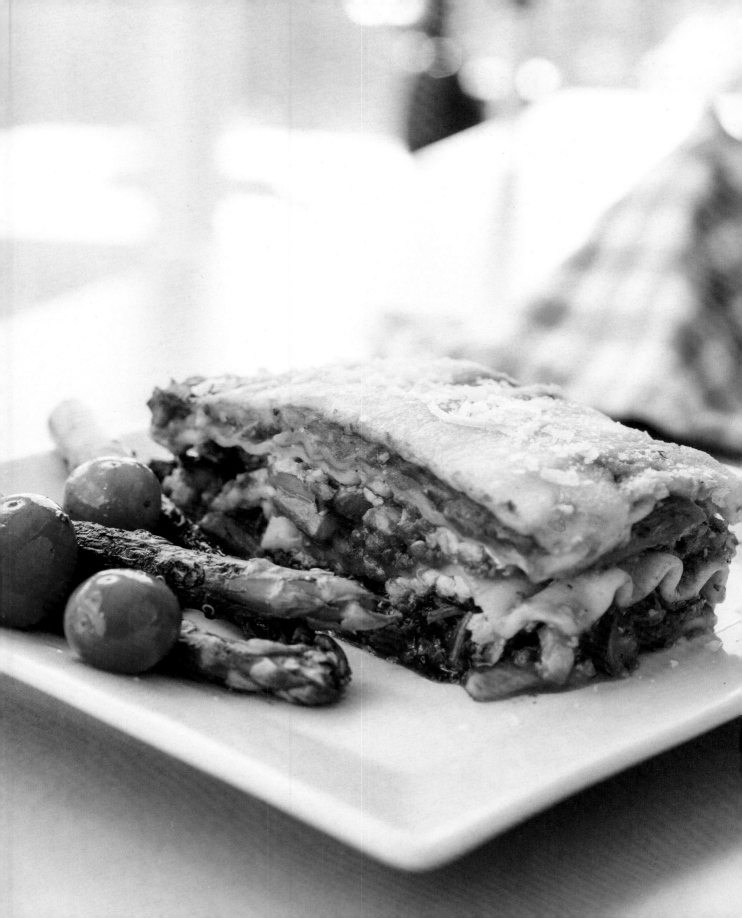

Carne asada

This steak is delicious in tacos. Prepare the steak according to the recipe, and add your choice of toppings. Carne asada also pairs well with mango cilantro slaw (page 148), cilantro lime rice (page 144), black bean soup (page 84), and black bean and corn salsa (page 98).

SHOPPING LIST: Skirt steak, fresh cilantro, limes, low-sodium soy sauce, Maggi's seasoning

CHECK FOR: Garlic, olive oil, sugar, salt

NUTRITIONAL ANALYSIS PER SERVING (3 OUNCES STEAK): 340 calories, 24 g fat, 6 g saturated fat, 26 g protein, 9 g carbohydrates, 1 g fiber, 353 mg sodium

1 pound skirt steak
2 tablespoons finely minced garlic
2 tablespoons finely minced fresh cilantro
2 limes
¼ cup low-sodium soy sauce
¼ cup olive oil
1 tablespoon Maggi's seasoning
1 tablespoon granulated sugar
¼ teaspoon salt

Clean and trim excess fat and tissue from skirt steak. (Note: You may need to cut it down to a size that fits your grill or cast iron skillet if it doesn't lie flat in the pan).

Apply pressure to the limes, rolling back and forth to loosen the fibers to make it easier to squeeze out the juice. In a large bowl, juice the limes. Add the garlic, cilantro, soy sauce, oil, Maggi's seasoning and sugar and combine.

Place the steak in the marinade; cover and let sit in the refrigerator at least 4 hours or overnight.

Remove meat from refrigerator and let sit at room temperature at least 20 minutes.

Heat a grill or cast iron skillet to high. Place the meat on the grill or skillet and cook about 2-4 minutes on each side. The meat should be medium-rare. Leave it on longer if you prefer it more well done.

Transfer meat to a cutting board. Cut the steak into 2-inch-thick pieces, then turn the steak and cut against the grain into small slices. Sprinkle with salt, and serve.

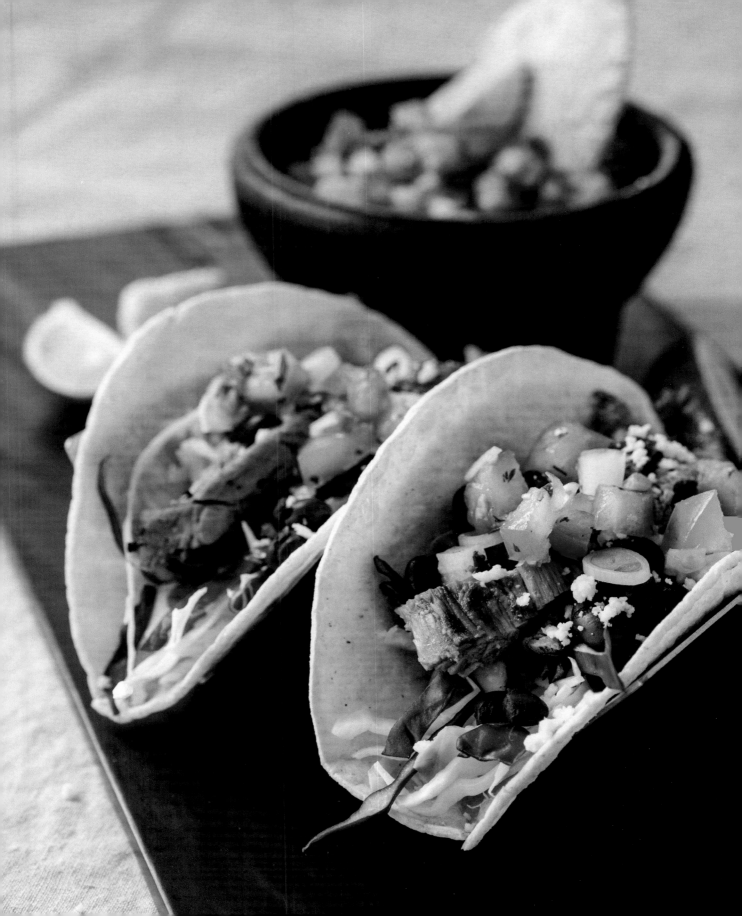

Swedish meatballs with quinoa

SERVINGS: 6 | ● ● ◖

Quinoa is used to reduce the amount of ground beef in the meatballs, if you're trying to reduce red meat in your diet. It adds bulk and provides protein. Quinoa also works as a gluten-free breadcrumb. Serve these meatballs with marsala sauce (page 210).

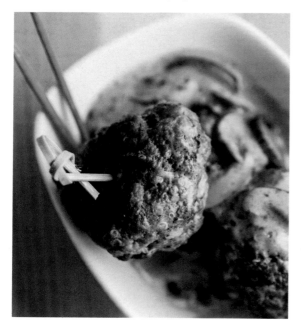

1 pound 95% lean ground beef
1 cup cooked quinoa
1 cup green chopped onion (about 6 onions)
1 large egg
½ cup ketchup
½ teaspoon kosher salt
½ cup panko breadcrumbs
¼ teaspoon ground black pepper
½ teaspoon garlic powder
1 tablespoon canola oil

Preheat oven to 350 F. In a medium-sized bowl, mix the lean ground beef with the cooked and cooled quinoa, green onions, egg, ketchup, kosher salt, panko, pepper and garlic powder. Make sure all ingredients are well combined.

Form the meatballs using a medium-sized scoop (about ¼ cup). Set them aside on a plate or a rimmed baking sheet.

Heat a nonstick sauté pan to medium-high heat. When hot, add the canola oil. Place meatballs in the pan, moving them around frequently to sear on all sides and develop a golden color.

Once meatballs are seared, return them to a cleaned baking sheet and bake in the oven until the meatballs reach an internal temperature of 160 F.

You can continue to cook the meatballs in the pan instead of finishing them in the oven. You'll want to turn down the heat to allow for more even cooking and to prevent burning, due to the limited amount of oil used.

SHOPPING LIST: Lean ground beef, quinoa, green onions, panko

CHECK FOR: Eggs, ketchup, kosher salt, pepper, garlic powder, canola oil

NUTRITIONAL ANALYSIS PER SERVING (1 MEATBALL): 240 calories, 8 g fat, 2 g saturated fat, 20 g protein, 21 g carbohydrates, 1 g fiber, 460 mg sodium

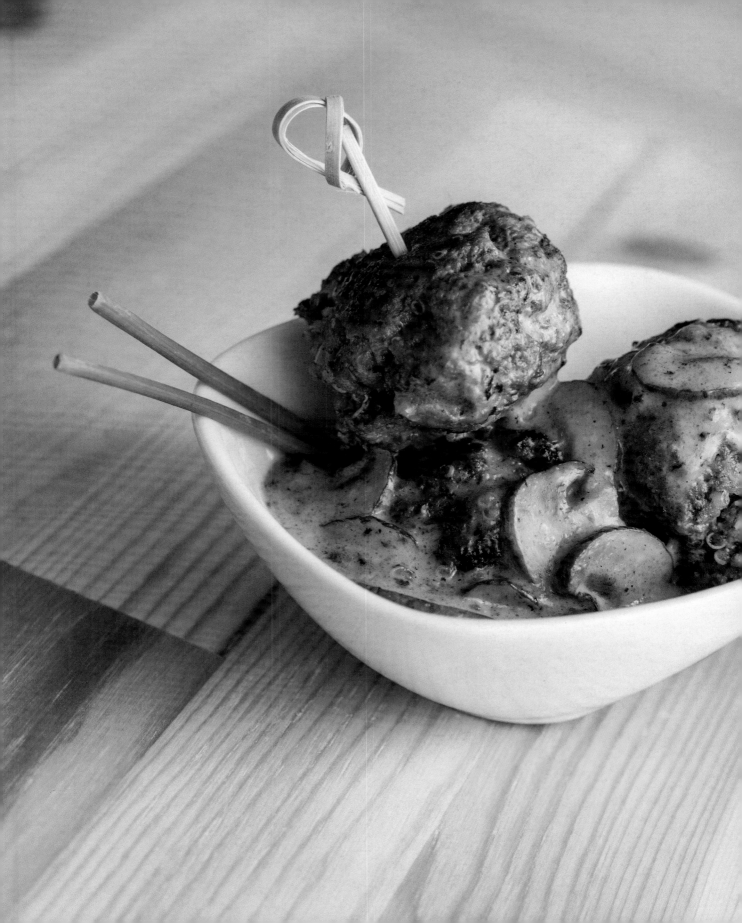

Shepherd's pie

SERVINGS: 6 | ◖●◖●

For a seasonal fall variation, try making this with mashed sweet potatoes instead of baking potatoes. Or add butternut squash, chopped small, to the vegetable filling.

½ cup diced onions
½ cup diced carrots (pea-size)
1 teaspoon olive oil
1 pound 95% lean ground beef
½ pound ground turkey breast
1 tablespoon tomato paste
½ teaspoon kosher salt
¼ teaspoon ground black pepper
1 teaspoon finely chopped fresh rosemary
1 teaspoon finely chopped fresh thyme
2 cups chicken stock
½ cup frozen peas, thawed
½ cup frozen corn, thawed
2 russet potatoes, washed and cut into small
    chunks
1 cup skim milk
¼ teaspoon kosher salt
1 tablespoon unsalted butter

Gather and prepare the ingredients. Set a medium pot of water with cut potatoes over high heat; cover and heat to boiling.

While potatoes are cooking, heat a large sauté pan to medium heat. Add oil to the pan and sauté the onions and carrots approximately 5-8 minutes or until tender.

Add the ground beef and ground turkey, stirring frequently to break up the meat. Add tomato paste, salt, pepper, rosemary and thyme. Then add the chicken stock, reduce the heat to medium and simmer 10 minutes.

Add the peas and corn, and cook about 10 minutes until most of the stock is absorbed or cooked off. Transfer the mixture to a casserole dish.

Once the potatoes are boiled and soft, drain and place them back on the stove over medium heat. Add the skim milk, salt and butter. Mash potatoes until smooth using an electric mixer or a potato masher. Spread the mashed potatoes on top of the meat mixture.

Cover and bake 15 minutes. Remove the cover and bake an additional 5 minutes until slightly brown around the edges. Serve hot.

SHOPPING LIST: Onions, carrots, lean ground beef, ground turkey breast, tomato paste, fresh rosemary, fresh thyme, chicken stock, frozen peas, frozen corn, russet potatoes

CHECK FOR: Olive oil, kosher salt, pepper, skim milk, unsalted butter

NUTRITIONAL ANALYSIS PER SERVING (1 PIECE): 290 calories, 9 g fat, 3.5 g saturated fat, 30 g protein, 23 g carbohydrates, 3 g fiber, 370 mg sodium

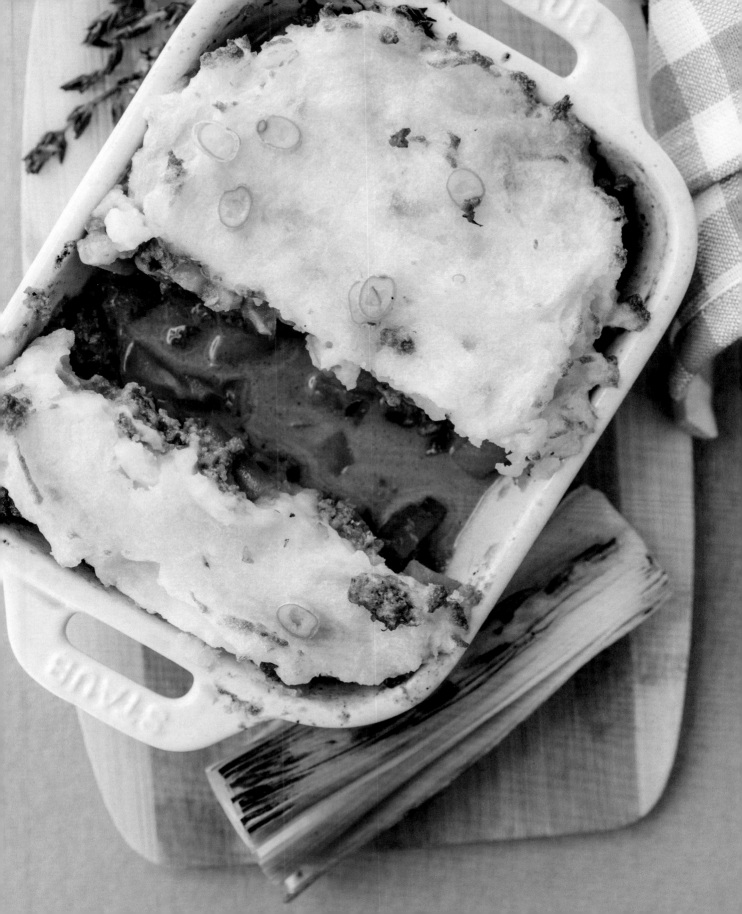

Southwest taco bowl

SERVINGS: 2 | ●●◖◖●●◖

To make a fresh cilantro lime dressing for this salad, combine the following in a food processor: the juice of 2 limes, ½ cup cilantro, 2 cups 1% cottage cheese, ¼ cup olive oil, ½ teaspoon salt, ½ teaspoon sugar, ¼ teaspoon black pepper and 1 clove garlic. Blend well.

SHOPPING LIST: Romaine lettuce, red bell pepper, green bell pepper, poblano peppers, sharp cheddar cheese, low-sodium black beans, ground turkey breast, lime juice, quinoa

CHECK FOR: Paprika, cumin, garlic powder, onion powder, salt, chili powder, oregano, cayenne pepper, cooking spray

NUTRITIONAL ANALYSIS PER SERVING (1 BOWL): 400 calories, 8 g fat, 3.5 g saturated fat, 36 g protein, 50 g carbohydrates, 16 g fiber, 650 mg sodium

2 cups roughly chopped Romaine lettuce (or whatever lettuce you have on hand)
1 cup chopped red bell pepper
1 cup chopped green bell pepper
2 poblano peppers, chopped
6 ounces ground turkey breast
2 teaspoons paprika
2 teaspoons ground cumin
½ teaspoon garlic powder
½ teaspoon onion powder
½ teaspoon salt
¼ teaspoon chili powder
¼ teaspoon oregano
¼ teaspoon cayenne pepper
¼ cup water
2 teaspoons lime juice
1 cup low-sodium black beans, rinsed
½ cup cooked quinoa
1 ounce sharp cheddar cheese, shredded

Gather and prepare the ingredients. Heat a medium sauté pan to medium heat and lightly spray with cooking spray. Add the peppers and sauté until soft, about 5 minutes; set aside and keep warm. Mix the seasonings together and set aside.

Heat another medium sauté pan to medium-high heat. Once hot, spray the pan with cooking spray and brown the ground turkey. Add the seasoning mixture, water and lime juice; cook until seasonings are well combined. Add the beans and quinoa and cook until warm.

Divide the lettuce into two bowls. Top with the vegetables, the cheese, and the turkey mixture. Serve with cilantro lime dressing.

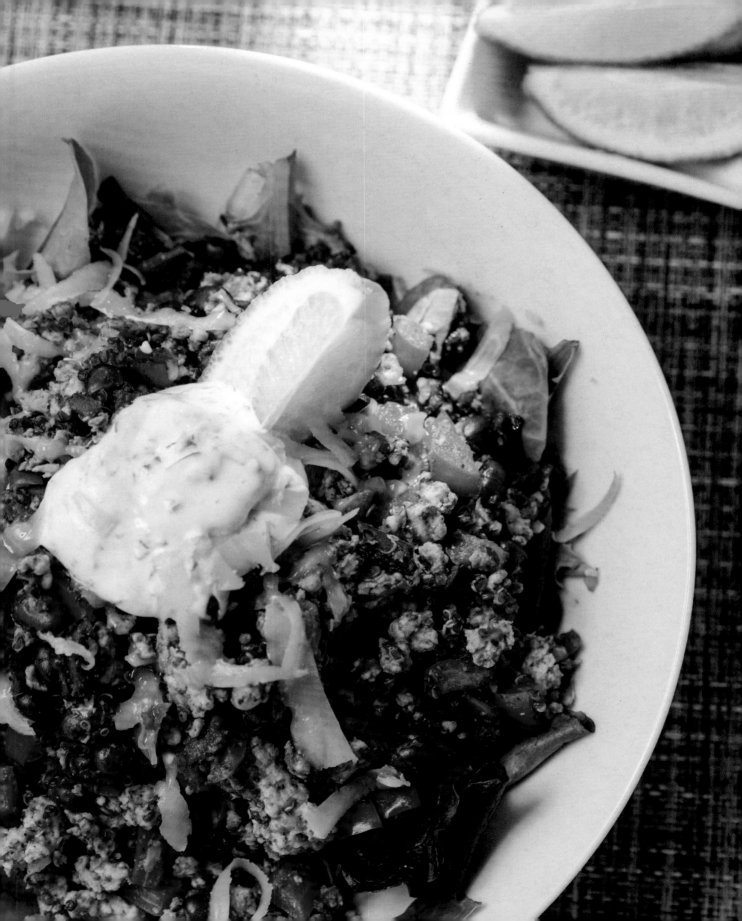

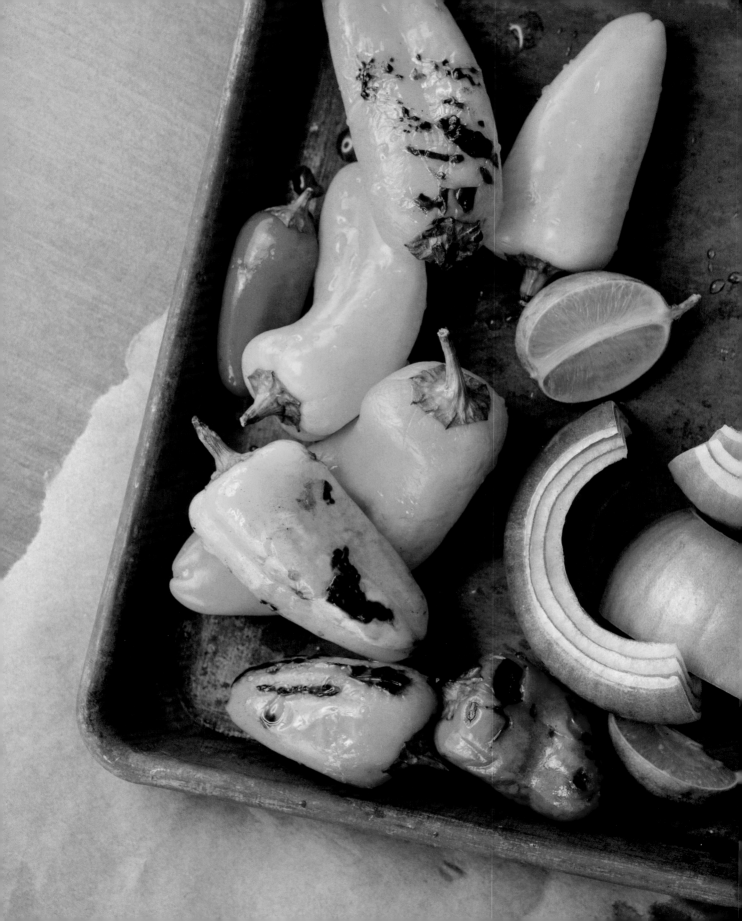

Vegetarian dishes

Double this recipe. Only makes 2.

Just OK Took forever ☆☆☆ to make.

Black bean burgers

3/17/22

Frying doesn't work. Try baking next time.

These burgers are a hearty vegetarian substitute for classic hamburgers. If you follow a vegetarian diet, make sure to add other plant protein sources to ensure you get a healthy dose of protein in your meals.

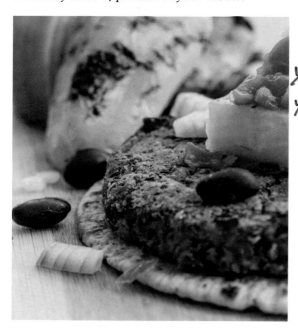

½ ¼ cup cooked quinoa
1 ½ cup finely chopped onion
½ cup black beans
2 1 ounce cheddar cheese, shredded
½ teaspoon garlic powder *2 ½ tsps*
1 ½ teaspoon onion powder
1 ½ teaspoon ground cumin
2 tablespoons finely chopped fresh cilantro
1 ½ teaspoon salt
½ ¼ teaspoon ground black pepper
1 egg white *2 egg whites*
½ ¼ cup panko breadcrumbs (to be used if mixture is too wet)
2 whole-wheat buns or whole-wheat tortillas
Put on flour tortillas

SHOPPING LIST: Black beans, onion, quinoa, cheddar cheese, fresh cilantro, panko, whole-wheat buns or tortillas

CHECK FOR: Garlic powder, onion powder, cumin, salt, pepper, eggs, cooking spray

NUTRITIONAL ANALYSIS PER SERVING (1 BURGER): 220 calories, 6 g fat, 3 g saturated fat, 12 g protein, 30 g carbohydrates, 6 g fiber, 480 mg sodium

Cook the quinoa. Chop the onion in a food processor or very fine with a knife. Spray cooking spray on a grill or medium sauté pan and heat to medium heat.

In a small bowl, mash the black beans and mix with the quinoa, cheese, onion, garlic powder, onion powder, cumin, cilantro, salt, pepper and egg white. Form the mixture into two patties. If the mixture seems too wet, add the panko.

Place the patties on the grill or in the pan and cook approximately 5 minutes on each side or until they reach an internal temperature of 140 F. Remove from heat and allow patties to rest until they reach a temperature of 145 F.

Place patties on the buns or tortillas and serve with your choice of condiments.

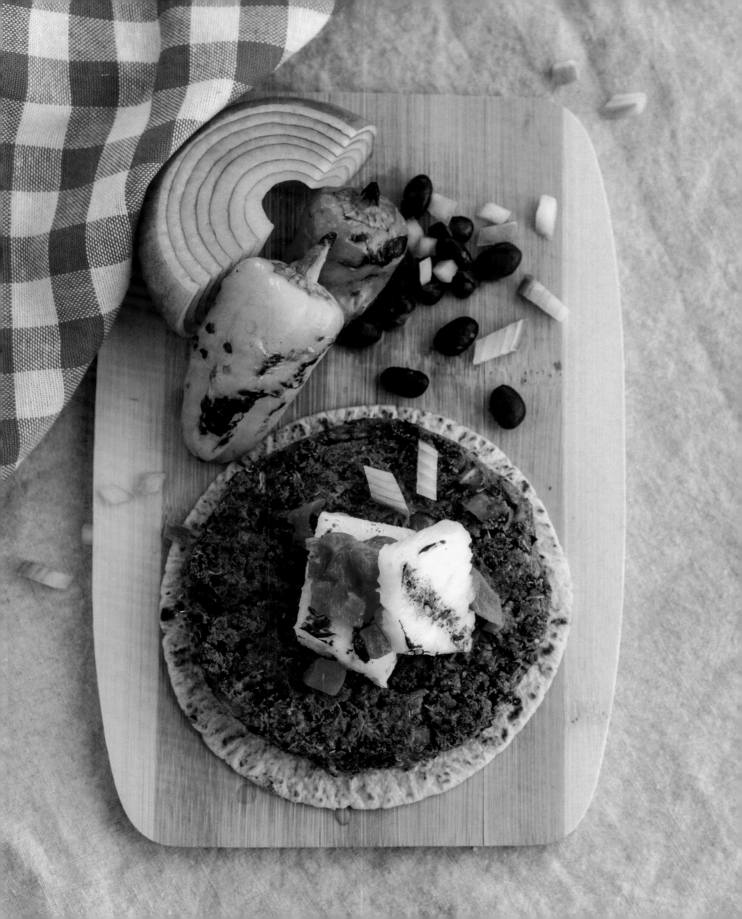

Black bean quesadillas

SERVINGS: 6 |

If you'd like to add meat, this quesadilla recipe works well with grilled chicken, shrimp or other lean meats.

SHOPPING LIST: Reduced-sodium black beans, zucchini, red onion, frozen sweet corn, fresh cilantro, sharp cheddar cheese, Tabasco sauce, whole-wheat tortillas

CHECK FOR: Cumin, salt, pepper, cooking spray

NUTRITIONAL ANALYSIS PER SERVING
(2 SLICES): 330 calories, 8 g fat, 3.5 g saturated fat, 17 g protein, 52 g carbohydrates, 10 g fiber, 640 mg sodium

3/14/2022
Awesome! Sauteed the veggies. Need to remember to melt cheese on top. ★★★★★

2 ¼ cups reduced-sodium black beans
1 ½ cups finely diced zucchini
1 cup finely diced red onion
1 ½ cups diced bell peppers, any color
⅓ cup chopped fresh cilantro
¾ cup shredded sharp cheddar cheese
1 ½ teaspoons ground cumin
¾ teaspoon salt
Pinch of ground black pepper
⅓ teaspoon Tabasco sauce
3 (12-inch) whole-wheat tortillas

Preheat oven to 350 F. Drain and rinse beans in a colander and place in a large bowl. Thaw corn in a colander under running water.

In a large bowl, combine the beans, zucchini, onion, corn, cilantro, cheese, cumin, salt, pepper and Tabasco sauce.

Heat a large nonstick sauté pan to medium heat. Coat with cooking spray. Place a tortilla in the pan for about 1 minute to warm. Place a third of the bean mixture on one side of the tortilla and fold the tortilla over to cover. Cook 1-2 minutes, then flip and cook another 1-2 minutes.

Remove from heat and place on a baking sheet. Repeat with the other tortillas. Bake 5-8 minutes or until the cheese has completely melted.

Cut each quesadilla into 4 slices. Serve with pico de gallo (page 203) and light sour cream.

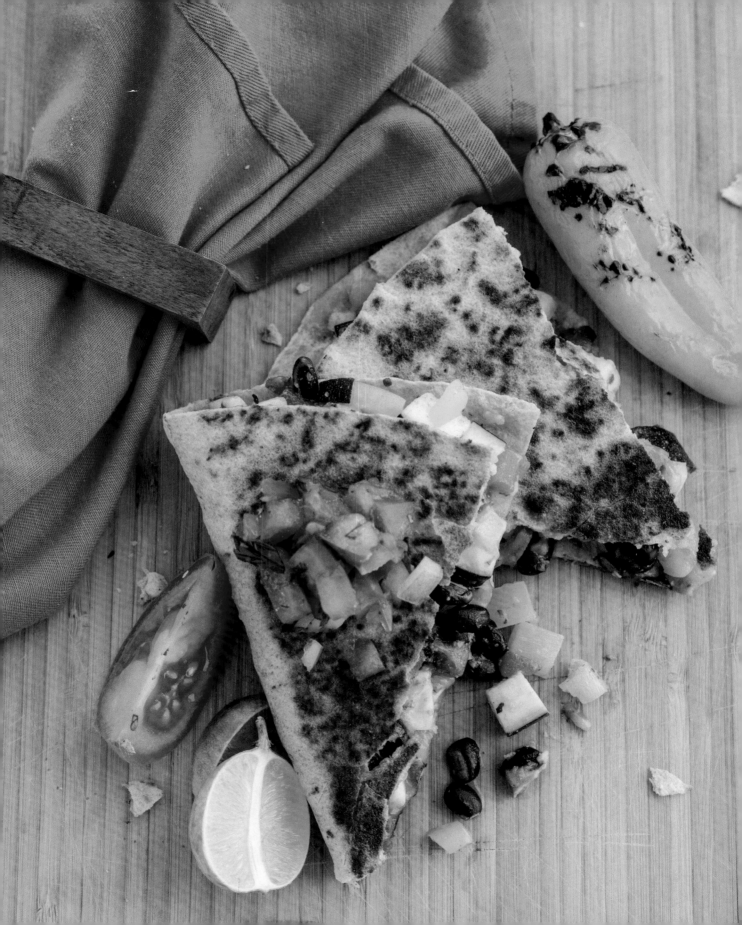

Edamame pad thai

SERVINGS: 4 |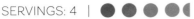

The vegetables in this recipe can be swapped out for other favorites or what you have on hand. Keep in mind that if you use a different vegetable, you may need to vary when it's added to the cooking process to avoid over- or undercooking it.

4 ounces uncooked rice noodles
2 cups broccoli florets
1 cup sliced red bell pepper
4 green onions, sliced thin
1 cup bean sprouts
4 cloves garlic, minced
1 teaspoon minced fresh ginger
4 cups edamame, shelled
4 tablespoons chopped unsalted peanuts
4 tablespoons chopped fresh cilantro

PAD THAI SAUCE
1 teaspoon chili paste
1 ½ tablespoons fish sauce
1 teaspoon low-sodium soy sauce
3 tablespoons brown sugar
3 tablespoons rice wine vinegar
2 tablespoons peanut butter
2 tablespoons water

Fill a medium soup pot with water and bring it to a boil. While waiting for the water to boil, place the pad thai sauce ingredients in a blender. Mix until well blended and smooth.

Cook the rice noodles in the pot according to package directions; stir frequently. Drain, rinse and set aside.

Heat a large nonstick sauté pan to medium heat. Once hot, add the red bell peppers, broccoli, onions and bean sprouts and sauté 2-3 minutes, moving them around quickly. Add the garlic, ginger and edamame, and cook an additional 1 minute.

Once vegetables are nearly cooked, add the rice noodles and ½ cup of pad thai sauce. Cook until the noodles are warmed through.

Serve hot, topped with chopped peanuts and cilantro.

SHOPPING LIST: Rice noodles, edamame, broccoli, red bell pepper, green onions, bean sprouts, fresh ginger, unsalted peanuts, fresh cilantro, chili paste, fish sauce, low-sodium soy sauce, rice wine vinegar

CHECK FOR: Garlic, brown sugar, peanut butter

NUTRITIONAL ANALYSIS PER SERVING (¼ RECIPE): 430 calories, 16 g fat, 2 g saturated fat, 27 g protein, 53 g carbohydrates, 12 g fiber, 620 mg sodium

Broccoli cheddar tofu cakes

When preparing the quinoa, make a large batch to use in other recipes later in the week or month. You can refrigerate the quinoa 5-7 days or freeze it up to 3 months.

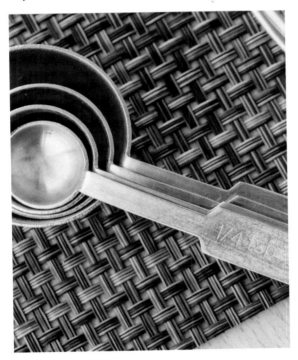

SHOPPING LIST: Broccoli, quinoa, extra-firm tofu, eggs, sharp cheddar cheese, panko

CHECK FOR: Garlic, onion powder, garlic powder, kosher salt, paprika, canola oil

NUTRITIONAL ANALYSIS PER SERVING (2 CAKES): 190 calories, 9 g fat, 3 g saturated fat, 13 g protein, 14 g carbohydrates, 1 g fiber, 260 mg sodium

3 cups broccoli florets, chopped small
2 tablespoons + 2 teaspoons uncooked quinoa
12 ounces extra-firm tofu
2 garlic cloves, minced
1 egg
1 teaspoon onion powder
1 teaspoon garlic powder
½ teaspoon kosher salt
¼ teaspoon paprika
2 ounces sharp cheddar cheese, shredded
½ cup panko breadcrumbs
1 ½ teaspoons canola oil

Preheat oven to 400 F. Steam the broccoli in the microwave or on the stovetop for 3 minutes. Cook the quinoa according to package directions.

Place the tofu in a food processor and blend until smooth. Add the garlic, egg, onion powder, garlic powder, salt and paprika. Mix well. Transfer the tofu mixture to a large bowl. Add the broccoli, cheese and quinoa.

Place the breadcrumbs in a medium bowl. Scoop ¼ cup of the tofu mixture and form into a ½-inch thick patty. Dip the patty in the panko and coat. Repeat with the remaining tofu mixture and panko.

Heat a large nonstick sauté pan to medium to medium-high heat; add oil. Cook the patties until golden brown on each side. Place them on a baking sheet and bake 5-10 minutes until heated through.

Pecan-crusted tofu

SERVINGS: 5 |

This is a great way to enjoy tofu. The tofu is hearty and flavorful and goes well with many other side dishes. Other nuts may be used in place of the pecans, such as walnuts or almonds; however, the overall flavor profile will change.

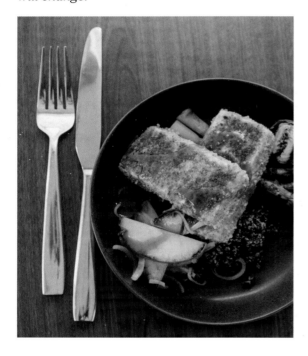

SHOPPING LIST: Extra-firm tofu, pecans, egg whites, maple syrup

CHECK FOR: All-purpose flour, brown sugar, kosher salt, Dijon mustard, honey, cooking spray

NUTRITIONAL ANALYSIS PER SERVING (1 PIECE): 340 calories, 13 g fat, 1 g saturated fat, 13 g protein, 41 g carbohydrates, 1 g fiber, 440 mg sodium

15 ounces extra-firm tofu, drained and dried
½ cup pecans
¼ cup all-purpose flour
2 tablespoons brown sugar
½ teaspoon kosher salt
½ cup egg whites, whisked

SAUCE
3 tablespoons Dijon mustard
6 tablespoons honey
3 tablespoons maple syrup

Preheat oven to 400 F, and lightly spray a baking sheet with nonstick cooking spray.

Cut the tofu into 5 planks. In a food processor, add the pecans, flour, brown sugar and salt and process until mixture has an even, finely chopped texture. Place mixture in a medium bowl and set aside. In a separate bowl, add the egg whites.

Set up a breading station as follows: the tofu first, then the egg whites, the pecan mixture, and the greased baking sheet. Dip tofu into the egg whites, then into the pecan mixture. Place on the baking sheet. Repeat until all tofu planks are well coated. Bake 15-20 minutes or until golden brown and crispy.

To make the sauce, mix the Dijon mustard, honey and maple syrup until smooth. Drizzle baked tofu with the sauce just before serving.

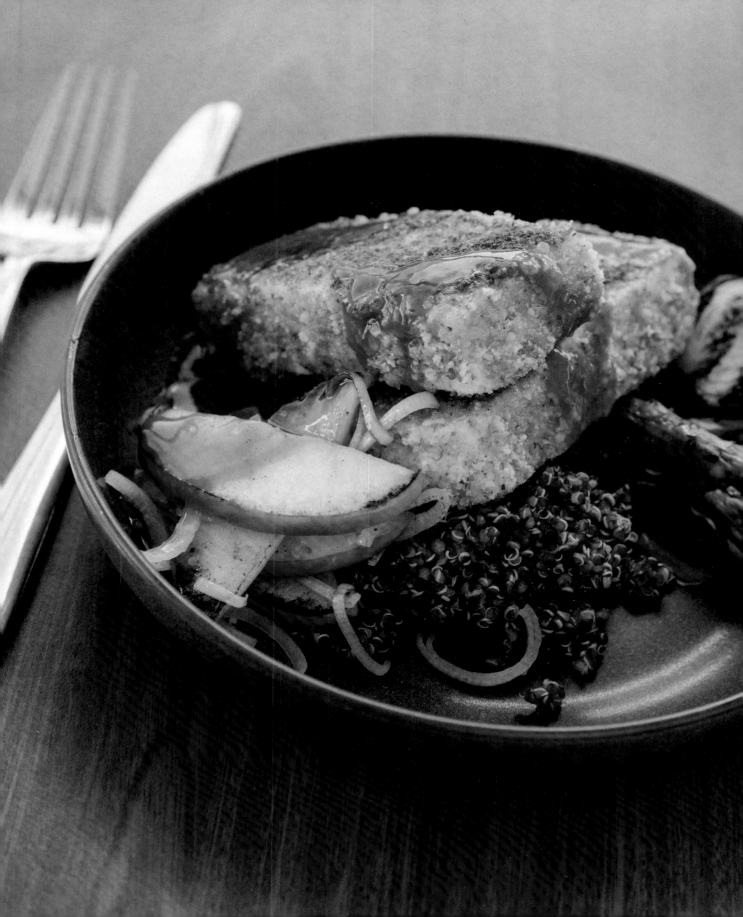

Thai peanut tofu stir-fry

SERVINGS: 4 |

Make sure to buy extra-firm tofu, as softer tofu will fall apart and scramble instead of remaining in cubes when you stir-fry it.

SHOPPING LIST: Extra-firm tofu, sesame oil, low-sodium soy sauce, rice wine or plain vinegar, scallions

CHECK FOR: Peanut butter, brown sugar, garlic, ginger, red pepper flakes, kosher salt

NUTRITIONAL ANALYSIS PER SERVING (¼ RECIPE): 350 calories, 22 g fat, 3.5 g saturated fat, 21 g protein, 20 g carbohydrates, 1 g fiber, 555 mg sodium

1 pound extra-firm tofu
2 tablespoons sesame oil
⅔ cup low-sodium soy sauce
¼ cup peanut butter
¼ cup brown sugar
2 tablespoons rice wine or plain vinegar
1 teaspoon minced garlic
2 teaspoons ground ginger
1 teaspoon red pepper flakes
½ teaspoon kosher salt
⅓ cup sliced scallions (about 1 bunch)

Drain and press the tofu to remove most of the moisture. Cut into cubes and set on a paper towel.

In a medium bowl or a blender, mix the soy sauce, peanut butter, brown sugar, vinegar, garlic, ginger, red pepper flakes and salt. Place the tofu in this sauce to marinate approximately 20 minutes.

Heat a large nonstick sauté pan to medium-high heat. Add the sesame oil. When hot, take the tofu cubes out of the marinade, shake off the extra liquid and place in the pan.

Shake the pan to loosen and turn the tofu so that the cubes brown on all sides. When tofu is lightly browned, add the marinade and cook together approximately 1 minute or until slightly thickened. Top with sliced scallions.

Serve over vegetables, such as bell pepper slices, and Asian noodles or rice.

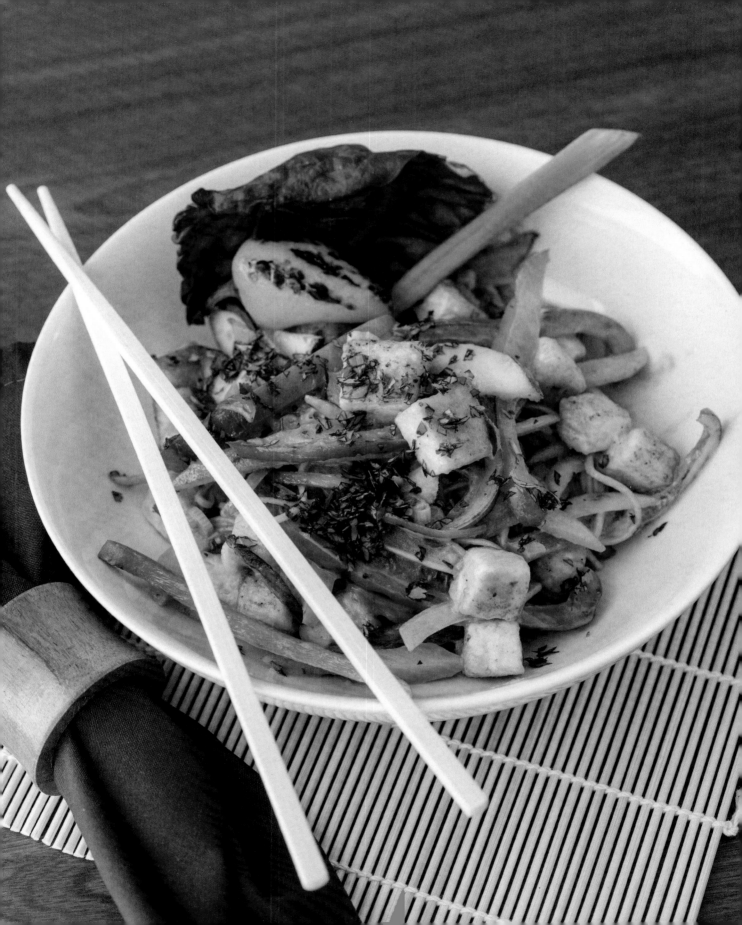

Spinach and Gruyère soufflé

SERVINGS: 4 |

To make a whole new type of soufflé, all you need to do is change the cheese used. You might try smoked gouda, extra sharp cheddar, Asiago or fontina.

3 egg whites
½ teaspoon unsalted butter
½ cup panko breadcrumbs
6 cups fresh spinach, stems removed
2 cups chopped cremini mushrooms
⅛ teaspoon salt
⅛ teaspoon ground black pepper
1 ½ tablespoons cornstarch
1 ⅓ cups skim milk
¼ cups Gruyère cheese
Pinch ground nutmeg

Preheat oven to 400 F. Lightly spray four 8-ounce ramekins with nonstick cooking spray. Sprinkle the ramekins with the breadcrumbs and place on a baking sheet.

Melt the butter in a medium sauté pan. Sauté the spinach and mushrooms, then season with salt and pepper.

Remove from pan and drain excess water from the spinach and mushrooms. When slightly cooled, chop any large pieces that remain and place in a mixing bowl.

In a medium saucepan, add the cornstarch and gradually whisk in the skim milk until smooth. Bring to a light boil over medium heat while whisking frequently. Reduce heat and stir in the Gruyère cheese. Pour the mixture over the cooked vegetables and season with nutmeg.

In a separate bowl, whip the egg whites with an electric mixer until stiff peaks form. Carefully fold the vegetable and milk mixture in with the egg whites, and place equal portions into the ramekins.

Reduce oven temperature to 375 F and place ramekins in the oven. Bake about 20 minutes or until the centers are firm and the tops slightly golden brown.

SHOPPING LIST: Panko, fresh spinach, cremini mushrooms, Gruyère cheese

CHECK FOR: Eggs, unsalted butter, salt, pepper, cornstarch, skim milk, nutmeg, cooking spray

---

NUTRITIONAL ANALYSIS PER SERVING (1 SOUFFLÉ): 200 calories, 6 g fat, 3 g saturated fat, 14 g protein, 22 g carbohydrates, 2 g fiber, 390 mg sodium

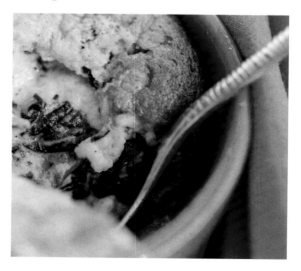

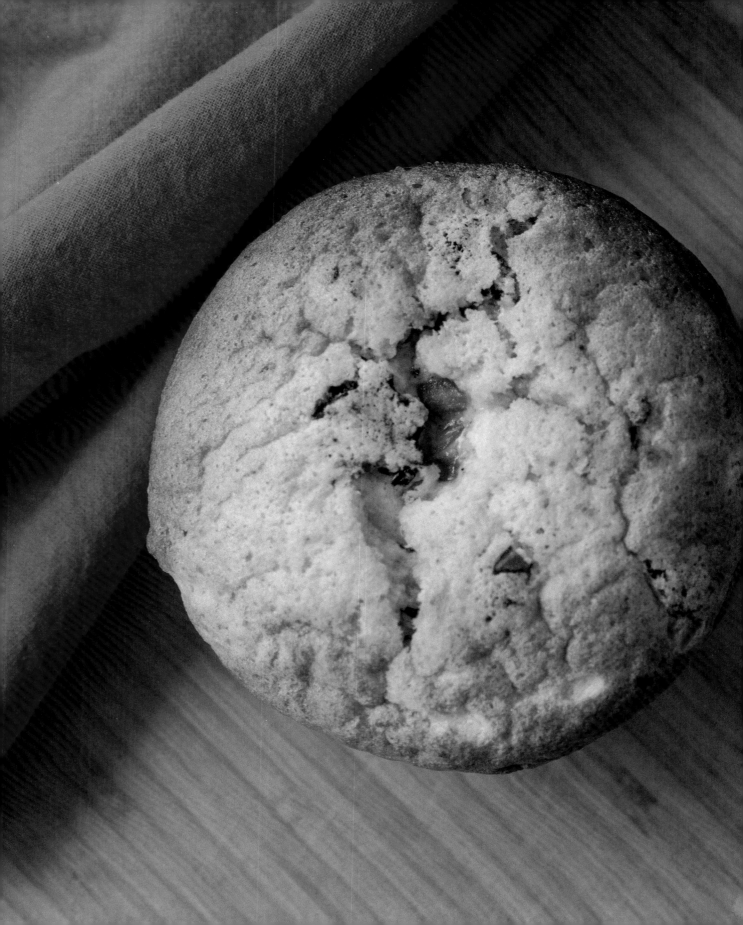

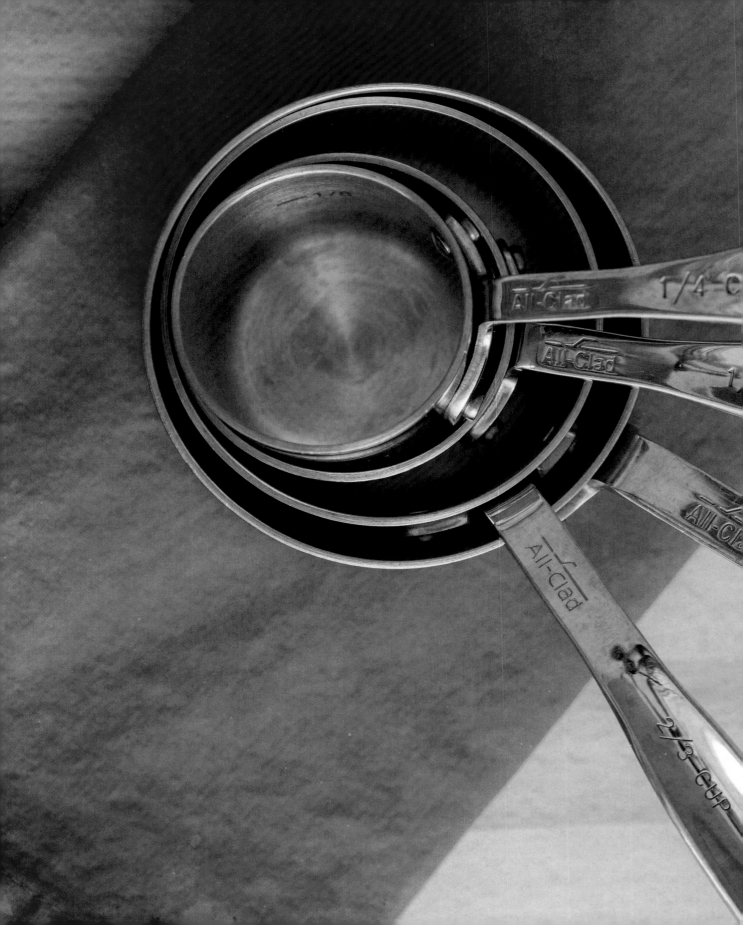

Sauces

Barbecue sauce

This barbecue sauce can be stored properly in the refrigerator for up to a month.

SHOPPING LIST: Onion, apple cider vinegar, unsweetened applesauce

CHECK FOR: Ketchup, honey, brown sugar, bay leaves, liquid smoke, cloves, chili powder, cayenne pepper, onion powder, garlic powder, paprika, pepper

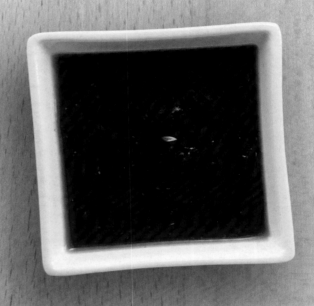

⅓ cup finely diced onion
4 cups ketchup
2 tablespoons honey
¼ cup brown sugar
½ cup apple cider vinegar
½ cup unsweetened applesauce
1 cup water
1 bay leaf
½ tablespoon liquid smoke
Pinch of ground cloves
½ tablespoon chili powder
⅛ teaspoon cayenne pepper
¾ teaspoon onion powder
¼ teaspoon garlic powder
¾ teaspoon paprika
Pinch of ground black pepper

Gather and prepare the ingredients. In a large pot, combine ingredients and bring to a boil. Lower the heat and simmer for 1 hour, stirring often.

Basil pesto

This recipe makes quite a bit of sauce. You can prepare it ahead of time. It also can be frozen and served with another dish.

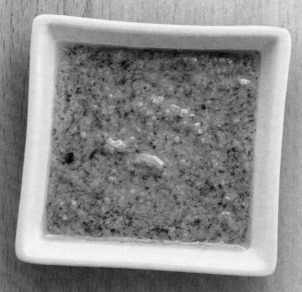

SHOPPING LIST: Fresh basil, pumpkin seeds, Parmesan cheese, lemon juice

CHECK FOR: Olive oil, garlic

2 cups fresh basil leaves
2 tablespoons pumpkin seeds
2 tablespoons fresh Parmesan cheese
1 tablespoon olive oil
1 tablespoon minced fresh garlic
2 teaspoons lemon juice

Place all the ingredients in a food processor. Process until the ingredients are well blended and smooth.

Teriyaki sauce

You can store this sauce in an airtight container in the refrigerator up to 7 days.

SHOPPING LIST: Low-sodium soy sauce, rice wine (mirin)

CHECK FOR: Sugar, garlic powder, ginger powder, cornstarch

¼ cup low-sodium soy sauce
¼ cup rice wine (mirin)
2 tablespoons sugar
1 cup water
½ teaspoon garlic powder
¼ teaspoon ginger powder
2 tablespoons cornstarch
2 ½ tablespoons water

Heat a pan to medium heat and add the soy sauce, rice wine, sugar, water and spices. Stirring continuously, cook until the sugar dissolves and the mixture reduces to a glaze. You can add some cornstarch combined with water (cornstarch slurry) to create a thicker sauce. Remove from heat and serve.

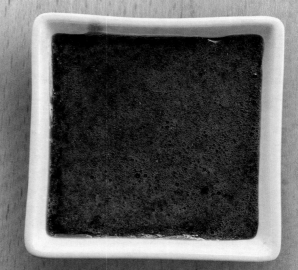

Pico de gallo

*Pickled jalapeños may be used in place of
fresh jalapeño peppers in this recipe*

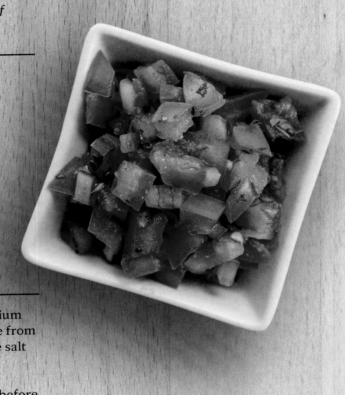

SHOPPING LIST: Roma tomatoes, onion,
jalapeño peppers, cilantro, lime

CHECK FOR: Garlic, sea salt

6 Roma seeded and diced tomatoes
⅔ cup diced red or white onion
¼ cup diced jalapeño pepper
⅔ cup finely chopped cilantro
4 cloves garlic, minced
1 lime
⅔ teaspoon sea salt

Place the first five ingredients in a medium
bowl. Cut the lime in half. Squeeze juice from
one of the halves into the bowl. Add the salt
and mix well.

Refrigerate the salsa for at least 1 hour before
serving.

Thai peanut sauce

This sauce is high in calories, so be aware of the extra calories in a large serving. If you want to make the sauce gluten-free, use tamari in place of low-sodium soy sauce.

SHOPPING LIST: Rice wine vinegar, low-sodium soy sauce or tamari, fresh ginger

CHECK FOR: Creamy peanut butter, cayenne pepper, garlic, red pepper flakes, onion powder, kosher salt, brown sugar

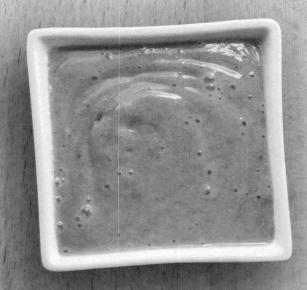

1 cup creamy peanut butter
½ cup rice wine vinegar
½ cup water
½ cup low-sodium soy sauce or tamari
¼ teaspoon cayenne pepper
1 ½ teaspoons minced garlic (about 2 cloves)
½ teaspoon red pepper flakes
½ teaspoon onion powder
Pinch kosher salt
¼ teaspoon minced fresh ginger
1 tablespoon brown sugar

Place the ingredients in a food processor or blender and blend until smooth and well combined.

Romesco sauce

Romesco sauce is traditionally made with a large amount of almonds. This version includes fewer nuts to lighten the calories, but it's not light on flavor! Try serving this robust sauce with fish, chicken, any lean meat, or even grilled and roasted vegetables.

SHOPPING LIST: Red bell peppers, whole blanched almonds, sun-dried tomatoes, sherry, fresh parsley

CHECK FOR: Garlic, olive oil, kosher salt, paprika

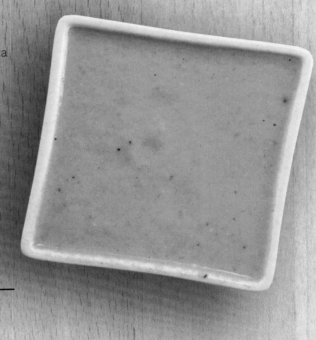

2 cups roasted red bell peppers (4 whole peppers, roasted, stems and seeds removed)
¼ cup whole blanched almonds
¼ cup sun-dried tomatoes
1 tablespoon minced fresh garlic
1 tablespoon sherry
¼ cup olive oil
¼ cup chopped fresh parsley
1 teaspoon kosher salt
½ teaspoon paprika

Place the ingredients in a food processor or blender and blend until smooth and well combined.

Serve cold or lukewarm.

Salsa verde

Raw tomatillos have a waxy, sticky texture that disappears when they are cooked.

SHOPPING LIST: Onion, jalapeños, tomatillos, fresh cilantro, lime juice

CHECK FOR: Sugar, salt

1 ½ pounds tomatillos
½ cup chopped onions
2 jalapeño peppers, chopped
½ cup chopped fresh cilantro
1 tablespoon lime juice
¼ teaspoon sugar
¼ teaspoon salt

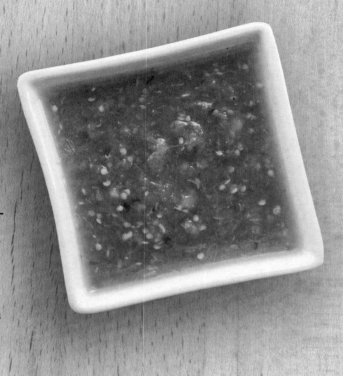

Preheat a grill or cast-iron skillet. Place the tomatillos on a grill or in a skillet and cook until the skin is slightly blackened.

Once the tomatillos have cooled, remove the skin. Cut the tomatillos in half and place them in a blender or food processor with the onions, jalapeños, cilantro, lime juice, sugar and salt. Blend until smooth.

Savory herb gravy

If you want to create a better mouthfeel for the gravy, add 1 tablespoon of butter. This, of course, adds calories, but might provide a more satisfying texture.

SHOPPING LIST: De-fatted low-sodium stock, shallot, peppercorns, fresh rosemary, fresh thyme, half-and-half

CHECK FOR: Bay leaves, cornstarch, salt, pepper, unsalted butter (optional)

4 cups de-fatted, low-sodium stock (chicken, vegetable or other)
1 bay leaf
1 shallot, chopped
4 peppercorns
1 tablespoon chopped fresh rosemary
1 tablespoon chopped fresh thyme
2 tablespoons cornstarch
2 ½ tablespoons water
¼ cup half-and-half
¼ teaspoon salt
Ground black pepper to taste
1 tablespoon unsalted butter, softened (optional)

Combine stock with the bay leaf, shallot, peppercorns, rosemary and thyme in a medium saucepan over medium-high heat. When the liquid reaches a boil, reduce the heat to low. Simmer uncovered until the stock is reduced in volume by about half (approximately 2 cups). This may take about 20 minutes over low heat. Strain out the herbs, bay leaf, shallot and peppercorns.

In a small, heavy-bottomed saucepan, bring the strained stock to a simmer. In a bowl, combine the cornstarch and water (cornstarch slurry). Add the half-and-half and cornstarch slurry to the stock, whisking constantly until a smooth gravy forms. Season with salt and pepper. Remove from heat.

Before serving, while the gravy is still warm, add the softened butter if you desire.

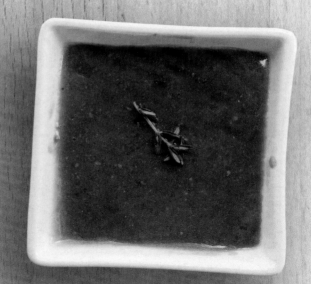

Lemon thyme sauce

It's best to add the cornstarch and water mixture a little at a time so the sauce doesn't get too thick. For additional flavor, add dill, tarragon or capers. You may use whole peppercorns in place of the ground pepper to create a less speckled sauce. Make sure to strain them out before serving.

SHOPPING LIST: Shallots, white wine, lemon juice, fresh thyme, peppercorns, half-and-half (optional)

CHECK FOR: Skim milk, bay leaves, unsalted butter, salt, pepper, cornstarch (optional)

¼ cup minced shallots
1 cup white wine
2 tablespoons lemon juice
1 ½ cup skim milk
1 bay leaf
1 tablespoon fresh thyme
¼ teaspoon whole peppercorns
2 teaspoons unsalted butter
⅛ teaspoon salt
⅛ teaspoon ground black pepper
2 tablespoons cornstarch mixed with ¼ cup cold water (optional)
3 tablespoons half-and-half (optional for color)

Heat a sauté pan to medium-high heat and sauté the shallots until they're lightly brown.

Add the white wine, thyme, peppercorns and bay leaf. Allow the wine to reduce by half. Add the lemon juice and continue to reduce.

Add butter, salt and pepper, then add the skim milk. Let the sauce return to medium-high heat. (The sauce may curdle due to the high acid content and the chemical action created when heat is applied. That's OK; a blender can fix it.)

If the sauce curdles, strain out the herbs, place the sauce in a blender and blend until the lumps are gone. Return to the pan.

If you would like the sauce to be thicker, add the cornstarch and water mixture and bring to a light boil. Add the half-and-half to give the sauce a creamier color.

Alfredo sauce

When serving Alfredo sauce with noodles, toss the noodles in the sauce to coat evenly. To enjoy the best flavor, serve immediately.

SHOPPING LIST: Reduced-fat cream cheese, fresh Parmesan cheese, white pepper

CHECK FOR: Olive oil, garlic, all-purpose flour, skim milk

1 teaspoon olive oil
2 tablespoons minced garlic
2 tablespoons all-purpose flour
2 ⅔ cups skim milk
¼ cup reduced-fat cream cheese
1 cup shredded fresh Parmesan cheese
1 teaspoon white pepper

Heat a medium sauté pan over medium-high heat. Add the olive oil and garlic to the pan and sauté 1 minute. Whisk in the flour and lower the heat to medium; cook 3-4 minutes.

Gradually add the milk, stirring until well blended. Cook until the mixture thickens, stirring constantly.

Stir in the cream cheese and cook until it melts, continuing to stir constantly. Turn off the heat and slowly add the Parmesan cheese and pepper. Stir until the cheese is melted into the mixture.

Marsala sauce

You can use any type of liquor or wine when making a pan sauce. Marsala sauce goes great with chicken breast or beef tenderloin, as well as pork tenderloin.

SHOPPING LIST: Shallots, mushrooms, fresh thyme, Marsala wine, veal or beef stock, fresh parsley, half-and-half

CHECK FOR: Garlic, salt, white pepper, cornstarch, butter (optional), cooking spray

2 tablespoons minced shallots
1 tablespoon minced fresh garlic
2 cups sliced mushrooms
1 teaspoon chopped fresh thyme
4 ounces Marsala wine
1 ½ cups veal or beef stock
1 tablespoon fresh parsley, chopped
½ teaspoon salt
Pinch white pepper
2 tablespoons half-and-half
¼ cup cold water
2 tablespoons cornstarch
1 tablespoon butter, cold or room temperature (optional for mouthfeel)

Heat medium saucepan to medium heat and spray with nonstick cooking spray.

Place the shallots in the pan and sauté approximately 2 minutes. Add the garlic, mushrooms and thyme and sauté another 2 minutes.

Add the Marsala wine and simmer approximately 1 minute. Add the veal or beef stock, parsley, salt, and pepper; simmer another 5 minutes until reduced by half.

Add the half-and-half. Mix the water and cornstarch (cornstarch slurry) and gradually add to the sauce for a thicker consistency. Add butter, if desired, for a creamier texture.

Marinara sauce

This sauce can be frozen into individual servings or stored in the refrigerator for at least a week. Use this marinara recipe for spaghetti, lasagna, pizza, chicken Parmesan, meatball subs, and more. You can omit the red wine if desired.

SHOPPING LIST: Onion, red wine, crushed tomatoes or tomato sauce

CHECK FOR: Garlic, olive oil, oregano, basil, sugar, salt, fennel, pepper

1 teaspoon olive oil
1 medium onion, chopped
3 garlic cloves, minced
1 cup red wine
5 cups crushed tomatoes or tomato sauce
1 tablespoon dry oregano
1 tablespoon dry basil
2 teaspoons sugar
¼ teaspoon salt
¼ teaspoon ground fennel
¼ teaspoon ground black pepper

Heat a medium saucepan to medium heat. Add the olive oil. Once the pan is hot, add the onion. Stir quickly for approximately 2 minutes. Add garlic and stir for 1 minute.

Add the wine and let mixture reduce by half. Add remaining ingredients. Stir and simmer on very low heat 15-20 minutes.

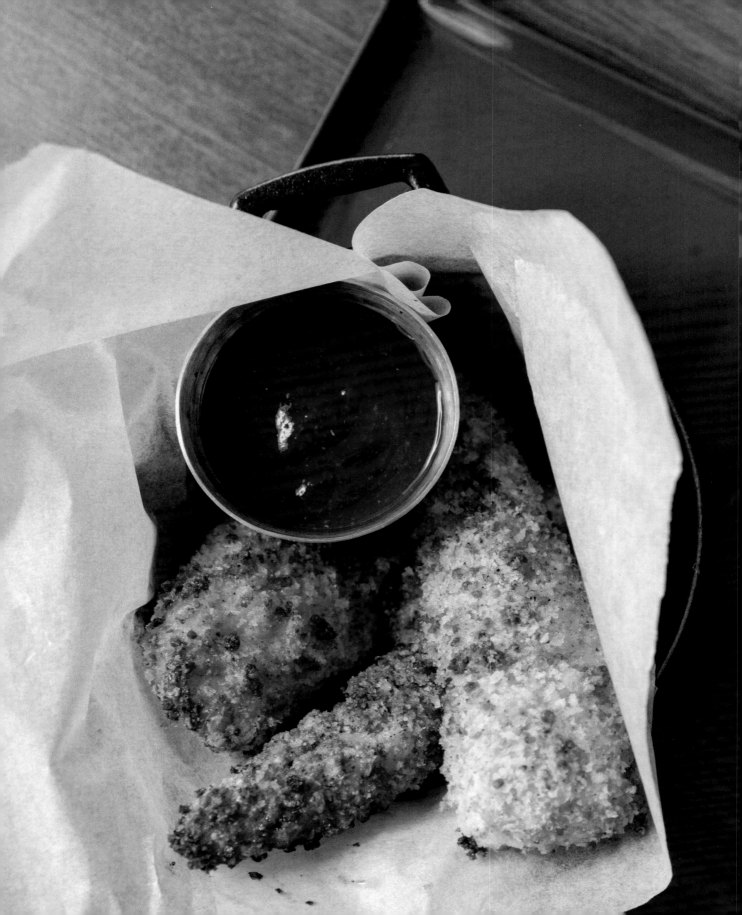

Kid-friendly foods

Baked macaroni and cheese

Other vegetables such as cauliflower, butternut squash, carrots, green beans or zucchini can be substituted for the broccoli. If children struggle with textures or types of vegetables, you can disguise veggies such as carrots and cauliflower by cooking them ahead of time and then puréeing with the cheese sauce.

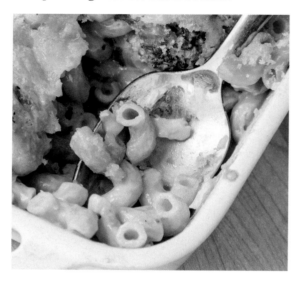

SHOPPING LIST: Whole-wheat or multigrain elbow pasta, reduced-fat cream cheese, sharp cheddar cheese, broccoli, panko (optional), fresh parsley (optional)

CHECK FOR: Skim milk, kosher salt, butter (optional)

NUTRITIONAL ANALYSIS PER SERVING (1 CUP): 260 calories, 11 g fat, 6 g saturated fat, 12 g protein, 29 g carbohydrates, 3 g fiber, 370 mg sodium

1 cup dry whole-wheat or multigrain elbow pasta
1 cup skim milk
3 tablespoons reduced-fat cream cheese
4 ounces sharp cheddar cheese, shredded
½ teaspoon kosher salt
4 cups broccoli, cut into bite-sized florets (or frozen broccoli florets, cooked)
½ cup panko breadcrumbs (optional)
¼ cup fresh chopped parsley (optional)
2 teaspoons butter, melted (optional)

Preheat oven to 375 F. In a medium to large saucepan, bring water to a boil. Add pasta and stir.

Cook pasta until soft but with a little crunch (about 2 minutes less than recommended cooking time). Strain the pasta and leave in strainer.

In the same saucepan, add the milk, cream cheese, cheddar cheese and salt, stirring constantly. Heat until the cream cheese melts and mixes in.

Return the drained pasta to the saucepan. Mix thoroughly and add the broccoli.

Transfer the macaroni mixture to a casserole dish. For a crunchy crust on top, sprinkle it with the optional mixture of the panko, parsley and butter. Place the casserole dish in oven and bake 15 minutes.

Remove from the oven and serve.

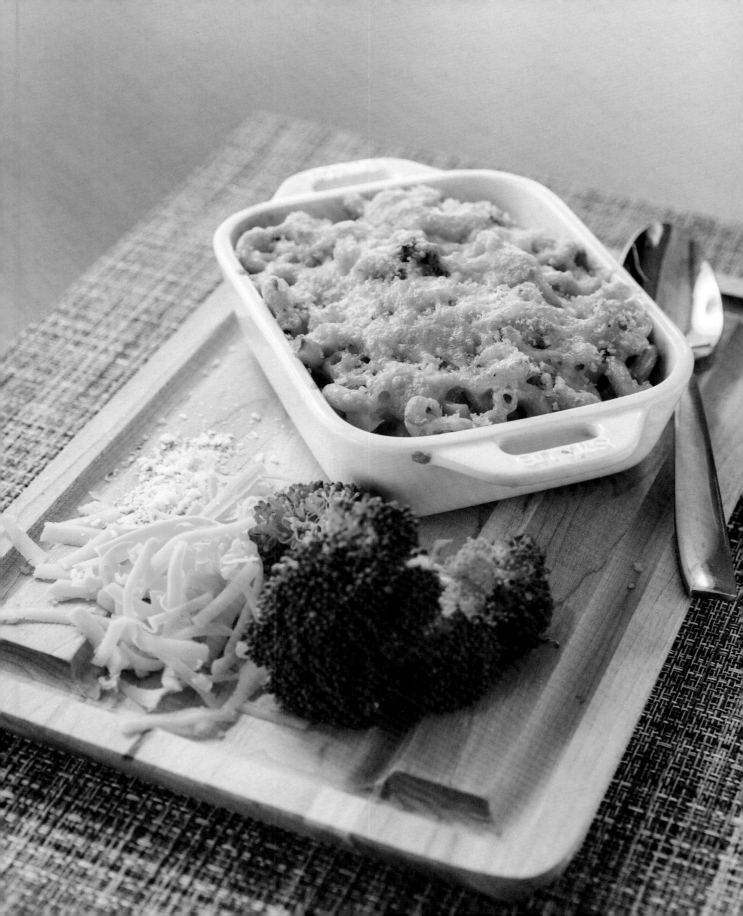

Crispy chicken tenders

Cornflakes gives these chicken tenders the true look of fried chicken. If you don't have yogurt, mix together ½ cup milk and one egg instead. Be sure to use a thermometer to check the doneness of your chicken tenders. Depending on the thickness of your chicken, some tenders can be done before others.

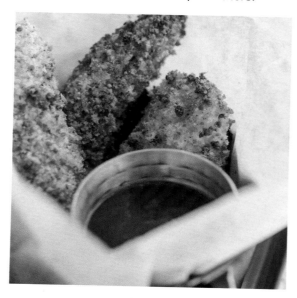

SHOPPING LIST: Boneless skinless chicken breasts, fat-free plain yogurt, cornflakes

CHECK FOR: All-purpose flour, kosher salt, garlic powder, onion powder, paprika, pepper, parchment paper, cooking spray

NUTRITIONAL ANALYSIS PER SERVING (2 TENDERS): 280 calories, 3 g fat, 0.5 saturated fat, 31 g protein, 29 g carbohydrates, 1 g fiber, 430 mg sodium

8 ounces boneless, skinless chicken breasts, cut into 1-ounce tenders
1 cup fat-free plain yogurt
2 cups cornflakes, crushed
½ cup all-purpose flour
½ teaspoon kosher salt
1 teaspoon garlic powder
1 teaspoon onion powder
1 teaspoon paprika
¼ teaspoon ground white pepper (ground black pepper also will work)

Preheat oven to 450 F. Line a baking sheet with parchment paper or spray it with cooking spray.

Remove all visible fat from the chicken and cut each breast into strips.

Place yogurt in a medium bowl. In a separate bowl, combine the crushed cornflakes, flour, salt, garlic powder, onion powder, paprika and white pepper.

Dip the chicken tenders in the yogurt. Then toss them in the seasoned cornflakes mixture to coat. Shake off excess cornflakes and lay the pieces out on the baking sheet.

Lightly spray the chicken tenders with olive oil or another cooking spray to help them brown. Bake approximately 15-20 minutes, until the tenders are slightly firm to the touch and reach an internal temperature of 165 F.

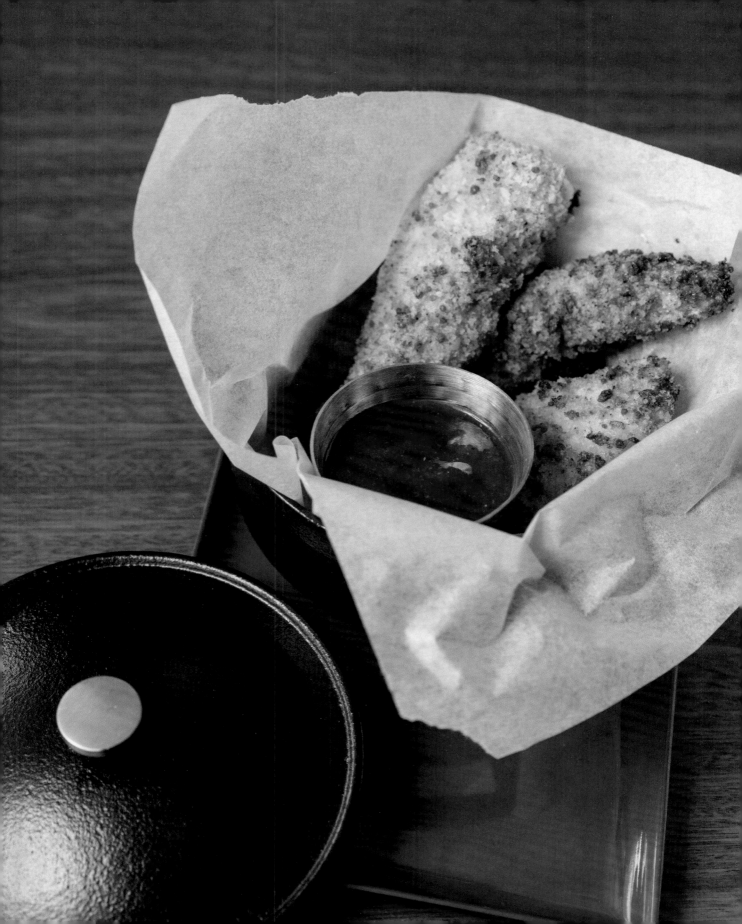

Cheesy polenta cups

SERVINGS: 16 |

These polenta cups are so versatile — easy finger foods for kids or nicely plated for a dinner party. You can make them even healthier by adding cooked vegetables such as cauliflower rice or even puréed cauliflower. The recipe makes a lot, so freezing the leftovers is another great way to have "emergency meals" ready for hungry children!

SHOPPING LIST: Polenta, fresh rosemary, fresh thyme, sharp cheddar cheese

CHECK FOR: Salt

NUTRITIONAL ANALYSIS PER SERVING (1 CUP): 110 calories, 2.5 g fat, 1.5 g saturated fat, 3 g protein, 17 g carbohydrates, 1 g fiber, 170 mg sodium

6 cups water
2 cups corn polenta (grits, or coarse cornmeal)
2 tablespoons chopped fresh rosemary
2 tablespoons chopped fresh thyme
1 teaspoon salt
½ cup shredded sharp cheddar cheese

In a medium saucepan, bring the water to a boil. Once boiling, slowly pour in the polenta while whisking briskly. This prevents lumps in the polenta.

Continue to whisk frequently. Once the polenta absorbs the water and starts to look thick and creamy, add the salt, herbs and cheddar cheese.

Remove the saucepan from the heat and whisk until the cheese is melted and seasonings are incorporated.

Pour the mixture into muffin tins, and let the polenta cool and set up in the pan. Once cool, the cups should release easily with a fork.

To serve, warm the cups in a 375 F oven for about 15 minutes, or place in a toaster oven for about 5 minutes.

Vegetable lasagna roll-ups

SERVINGS: 6 |

Make this recipe your own. You can add browned chicken sausage to the vegetable mixture if you'd like. If you want to keep the recipe vegetarian, cube extra-firm tofu and combine it with the vegetables.

BASIL PESTO MAYO
1 cup fresh basil leaves
¼ cup pumpkin seeds
¼ cup fresh Parmesan cheese
3 cloves garlic
½ teaspoon kosher salt
1 cup reduced-fat mayonnaise

6 whole-wheat lasagna noodles
1 teaspoon olive oil
¾ cup chopped mushrooms
¾ cup chopped onions
1 tablespoon minced garlic
1 cup chopped zucchini
¾ cup chopped beefsteak tomatoes
½ cup part-skim ricotta cheese
¾ cup shredded mozzarella cheese
½ cup skim (or low-fat) milk
½ cup chopped red bell pepper

To prepare the basil pesto mayo, place the fresh basil, pumpkin seeds, Parmesan cheese, garlic and salt in a food processor and process until well-blended and fairly smooth. Add the mayonnaise and pulse until just blended. Refrigerate until ready for use.

Preheat the oven to 350 F. Boil the lasagna noodles according to package directions; drain and set aside. Meanwhile, prepare the vegetables and garlic.

In a large nonstick sauté pan, heat the oil. Add the mushrooms, onions and garlic and sauté about 3 minutes. Add the zucchini and tomatoes and sauté an additional 3-5 minutes, until tender. Remove from heat. Add the ricotta and mozzarella cheeses.

Coat a baking dish with cooking spray. Lay out the cooked lasagna noodles in the dish and lightly coat with cooking spray. Place ½ cup of the vegetable mixture at the end of each noodle, then roll up. Mix ¼ cup of the basil pesto mayo with ½ cup skim (or low-fat) milk and drizzle over the noodles.

Cover with parchment paper and foil, and bake approximately 25 minutes. Uncover and sprinkle with the chopped red bell pepper and some mozzarella cheese. Bake about 3 minutes until the cheese is melted.

SHOPPING LIST: Fresh basil leaves, pumpkin seeds, Parmesan cheese, whole-wheat lasagna noodles, zucchini, mushrooms, onion, beefsteak tomatoes, part-skim ricotta cheese, mozzarella cheese, red bell pepper

CHECK FOR: Garlic, kosher salt, reduced-fat mayonnaise, olive oil, skim milk, cooking spray

NUTRITIONAL ANALYSIS PER SERVING (1 ROLL-UP): 300 calories, 8 g fat, 4 g saturated fat, 14 g protein, 39 g carbohydrates, 5 g fiber, 300 mg sodium

Parmesan zucchini fingers

To help brown the zucchini, spray a little olive oil or cooking spray over each plank. Eggplant and yellow summer squash are great alternatives that can be used in place of the zucchini in this recipe.

SHOPPING LIST: Zucchini, panko, Parmesan cheese, marinara sauce

CHECK FOR: Eggs, garlic powder, onion powder, basil, oregano, kosher salt, pepper

NUTRITIONAL ANALYSIS PER SERVING (APPROX. 3 FINGERS): 230 calories, 4.5 g fat, 1.5 g saturated fat, 11 g protein, 35 g carbohydrates, 5 g fiber, 670 mg sodium

2 medium zucchini, cut into 3- to 4-inch planks
2 egg whites
2 tablespoons water
1 cup panko breadcrumbs
½ cup grated Parmesan cheese
1 teaspoon garlic powder
1 teaspoon onion powder
2 teaspoons dry basil
2 teaspoons dry oregano
½ teaspoon kosher salt
Ground black pepper
2 cups marinara sauce

Preheat oven to 425 F. Spray a baking sheet with cooking spray.

Mix egg whites in a medium to large bowl. Add 2 tablespoons water to thin out the egg mixture.

In another bowl, mix the panko, Parmesan cheese and seasonings. If the mixture is really chunky, place it in a food processor and process a few seconds to get a more even consistency.

Dip each plank into the egg white mixture, and then dredge in the panko mixture. Place on the baking sheet, making sure not to overcrowd each piece. (Air around each piece will help it brown and become crisp.)

Bake approximately 15-20 minutes or until golden brown. Serve with marinara sauce (page 211).

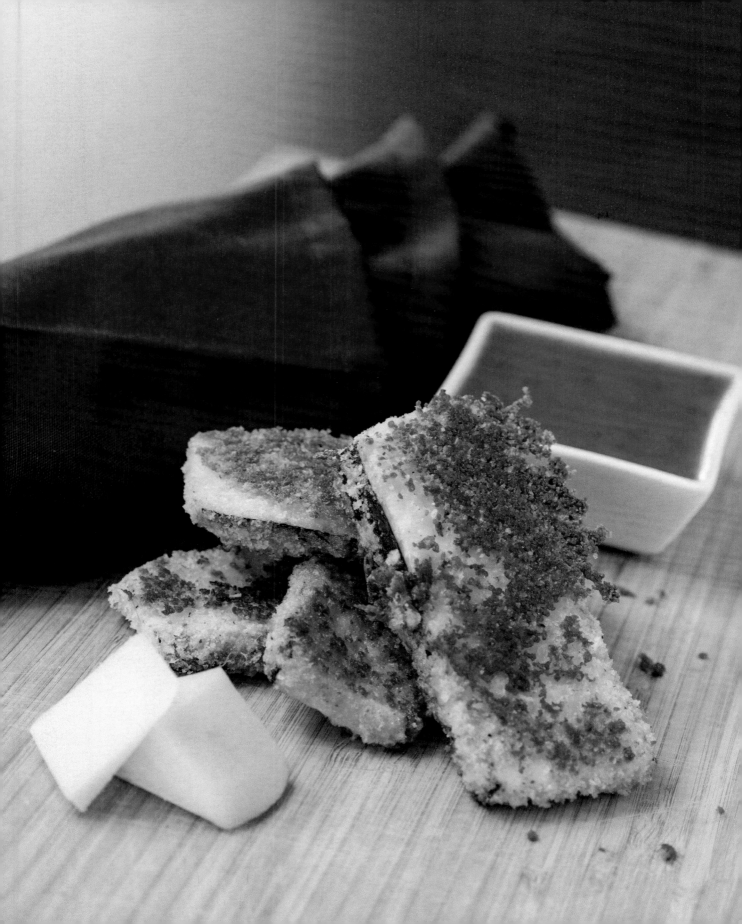

Pita pizza

SERVINGS: 1 |

If you prefer other toppings, simply replace those listed or remove the ones you don't care for. Try to include a variety of vegetables to get a variety of nutrients and color. Cooking for more than one? Make this recipe for four people using ½ cup each of mushrooms, bell pepper and feta, 1 cup each of red onion and marinara, and 1 ½ cups mozzarella cheese.

SHOPPING LIST: Whole-wheat pita, marinara sauce, button mushrooms, red onion, pineapple, bell pepper, part-skim mozzarella cheese, reduced-fat feta cheese, turkey bacon bits

CHECK FOR: Cooking spray

NUTRITIONAL ANALYSIS PER SERVING (1 PIZZA): 330 calories, 9 g fat, 4 g saturated fat, 17 g protein, 46 g carbohydrates, 8 g fiber, 680 mg sodium

1 (6-inch) whole-wheat pita
¼ cup marinara sauce
2 tablespoons sliced button mushrooms
¼ cup red onion
2 tablespoons pineapple
2 tablespoons bell pepper
3 tablespoons part-skim mozzarella cheese
2 tablespoons reduced-fat feta cheese
1 teaspoon turkey bacon bits

Preheat oven or toaster oven to 375 F. Lightly coat a baking sheet with cooking spray. Place pita on baking sheet.

Gather and prepare your ingredients. Spread the marinara over the pita. Add the vegetables and pineapple in an even layer. Top with the cheeses and bacon bits.

Bake 15-20 minutes in the oven. If using a toaster oven, cook 5-10 minutes.

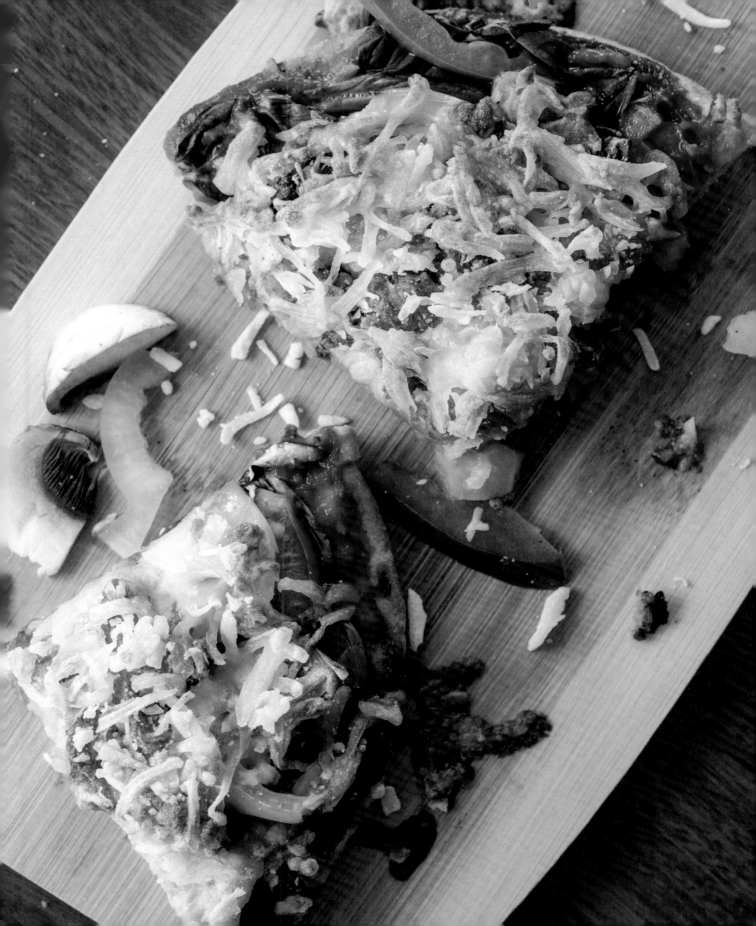

Broccoli macaroni bites

SERVINGS: 24 |

For easy frozen meals, prepare a batch of bites through the breading process and freeze them on a baking sheet. Once frozen, store in an airtight container in the freezer. Cook as many as desired for 20 minutes in a preheated oven.

SHOPPING LIST: Macaroni, broccoli, sharp cheddar cheese, pepper jack cheese, panko, Parmesan cheese

CHECK FOR: Kosher salt, garlic powder, eggs

NUTRITIONAL ANALYSIS PER SERVING (1 BITE): 120 calories, 7 g fat, 4 g saturated fat, 7 g protein, 7 g carbohydrates, 260 mg sodium

2 cups dry macaroni
4 cups broccoli, chopped into small florets
8 ounces shredded sharp cheddar cheese
8 ounces shredded pepper jack cheese
1 teaspoon kosher salt

BREADING
¾ cup panko breadcrumbs
½ cup grated Parmesan cheese
½ teaspoon garlic powder
¼ teaspoon kosher salt
1 egg

Preheat oven to 425 F. Lightly spray a baking sheet with cooking spray.

Cook macaroni in a large saucepan according to package directions, adding the broccoli florets about 5 minutes before the macaroni is done. Drain the pasta and broccoli. In a large bowl, add the pasta and broccoli and mix in the shredded cheeses and salt.

In a small bowl, add the panko, Parmesan cheese, garlic powder and kosher salt and combine. In another small bowl, add the egg and whisk.

Shape the macaroni mixture into balls, with each ball about ¼ cup in size. Press a little firmly on each ball to assure the contents stick.

Roll each macaroni ball in the egg mixture to coat it and then into the panko mixture. Place the ball on the baking sheet. Bake approximately 15 minutes, and serve hot.

Frittata muffins

These "muffins" are great for feeding kids — or yourself — on the go. Try them with different vegetables (bell peppers, mushrooms, onions, zucchini or poblano peppers) or cheeses (feta, pepper jack or mozzarella). Simply reheat the muffins in a toaster oven or microwave to serve throughout the week.

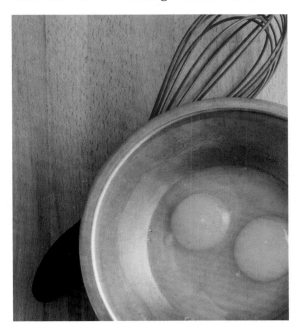

SHOPPING LIST: Spinach, bacon, sharp cheddar cheese

CHECK FOR: Eggs, kosher salt, pepper

NUTRITIONAL ANALYSIS PER SERVING (1 MUFFIN): 90 calories, 6 g fat, 3 g saturated fat, 8 g protein, 1 g carbohydrates, 1 g fiber, 250 mg sodium

6 cups spinach
6 egg whites
6 whole eggs
2 slices bacon, cooked and chopped very finely
½ teaspoon kosher salt
¼ teaspoon ground black pepper
1 cup shredded sharp cheddar cheese

Preheat oven to 375 F. Lightly spray a muffin pan with cooking spray and set aside.

Sauté the spinach over medium heat in a nonstick pan. Cook until it's wilted and its water has evaporated. If you're unsure whether its water has evaporated, drain the spinach in a strainer.

In a mixing bowl, whisk the eggs with the egg whites. Gradually add in the chopped bacon, salt, pepper and cheese.

Divide the cooked spinach between 12 muffin cups. Fill the muffin cups with the egg mixture, cover with foil and bake approximately 15-20 minutes. Check frittatas. If the egg mixture is fairly set, then place the muffin tin back in the oven uncovered for about 5 minutes.

Remove muffin pan from the oven. Use a fork or knife to gently remove the frittatas from the muffin cups. Serve immediately, or let cool and store in the refrigerator for 3-4 days and reheat.

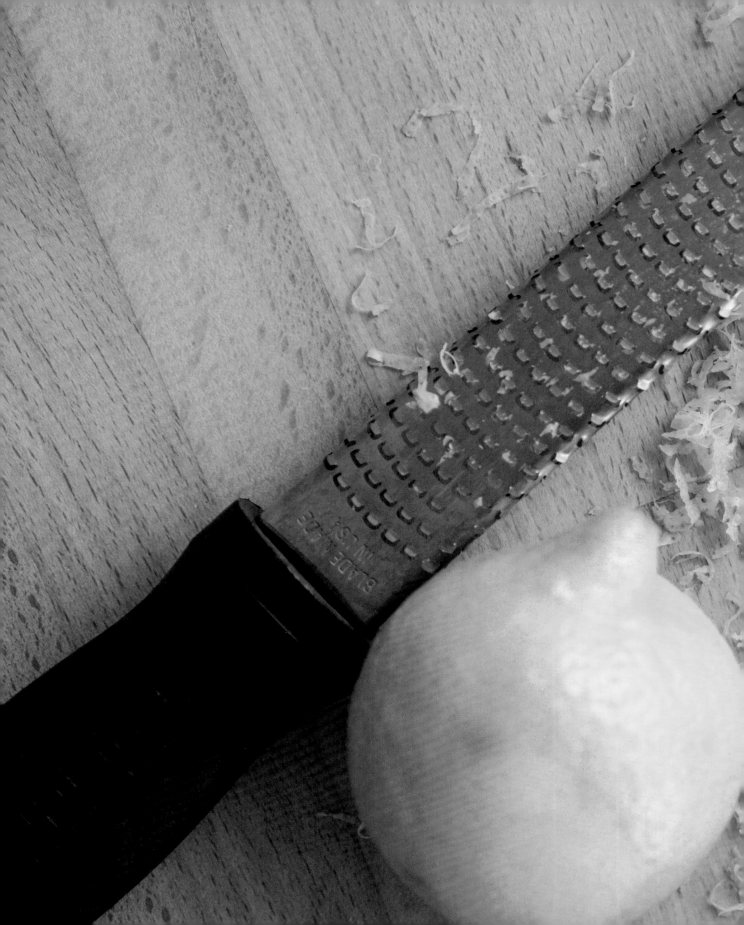

Desserts

Strawberry sorbet

The best way to use less sugar in a sorbet recipe is to use the ripest produce you can find. If out of season, frozen berries tend to be a better option than fresh. And don't skip the little bit of lime juice! If you're out of limes, try lemon juice, orange juice or pineapple juice instead.

4 pints fresh strawberries, sliced
1 cup fresh or frozen cranberries
1 cup sugar
2 cups water
2 tablespoons lime juice, fresh squeezed

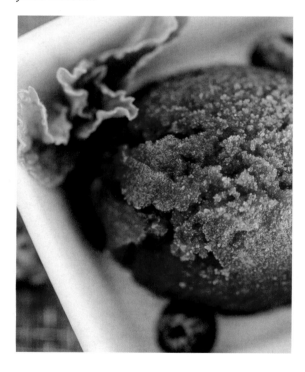

This dessert requires an ice cream maker. The night or day before, place the bowl of your ice cream maker in the freezer. You may want to freeze the container you'll use for storing the ice cream, too.

In a medium saucepan, warm the strawberries, cranberries, sugar and water until the sugar is dissolved.

Purée the strawberry mixture in a blender. To strain out the strawberry seeds, pour the blended liquid through a fine-mesh strainer. Mix in the fresh lime juice.

Cool the mixture in the refrigerator. Or to cool it down faster, place the mixture in a metal bowl, and set it on top of another bowl full of ice water. Stir occasionally.

Once the strawberry mixture is cool, turn your ice cream maker on and pour the mixture into the bowl. Within about 20 minutes, it will become thicker and almost slushy. Place the soft sorbet into a container with a lid and freeze at least 4 hours or overnight.

To portion this dessert, use a 1-ounce scoop, which equals about 2 tablespoons.

SHOPPING LIST: Strawberries, cranberries, lime

CHECK FOR: Sugar

NUTRITIONAL ANALYSIS PER SERVING (ABOUT 2 TABLESPOONS): 100 calories, 1 g protein, 2 g carbohydrates, 26 mg sodium

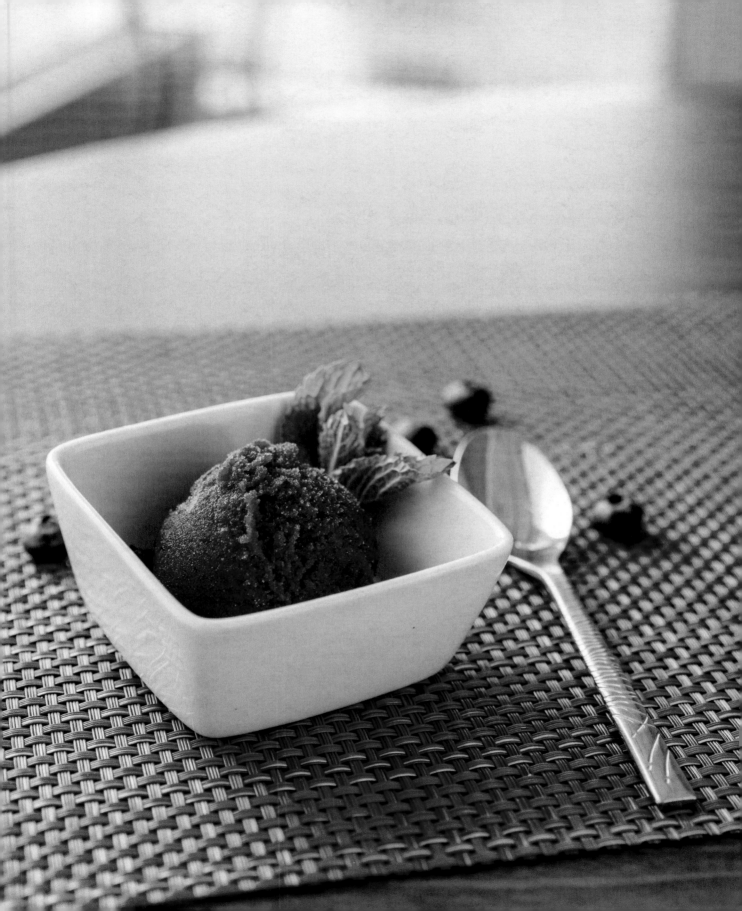

Lemon pudding cakes

SERVINGS: 6 |

To give these cakes a different flavor, you can substitute limes for the lemons. Replacing the lemons with an orange will give the pudding cakes a dreamsicle-like flavor.

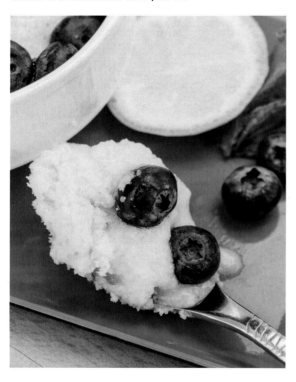

SHOPPING LIST: Lemons

CHECK FOR: Eggs, salt, sugar, skim milk, all-purpose flour, butter

---

NUTRITIONAL ANALYSIS PER SERVING (1 CAKE): 130 calories, 3.5 g fat, 1.5 g saturated fat, 4 g protein, 24 g carbohydrates, 120 mg sodium

2 medium lemons
2 eggs, separated
¼ teaspoon salt
¾ cup sugar
1 cup skim milk
3 tablespoons all-purpose flour
1 tablespoon butter, melted

Preheat oven to 350 F. Grease six 6-ounce custard cups or small ramekins. Zest the lemon peel to measure 1 tablespoon. Squeeze juice from lemons, to measure ⅓ cup. Set aside.

Using an electric mixer, beat the egg whites and salt at high speed until soft peaks form. Gradually add ½ cup sugar, beating until sugar completely dissolves and egg whites stand in stiff peaks. (Soft peaks will curl around if you turn a beater upside down, while stiff peaks hold their shape.)

In a large bowl, beat the egg yolks at medium speed with the remaining ¼ cup sugar until blended. Add the lemon zest and juice, milk, flour and butter. Beat until mixed well, scraping the bowl with a rubber spatula.

With a wire whisk or spatula, gently fold the beaten egg whites into the egg yolk mixture until barely mixed. Pour the batter into the custard cups or ramekins. Set the cups in a 9x13-inch baking pan and place on oven rack. Carefully fill the baking pan with boiling water to come halfway up the sides of the custard cups. Bake 40-45 minutes, until the tops are golden and firm. (The cakes will separate into a cake layer on top and a sauce layer underneath.)

Cool puddings in custard cups on a wire rack.

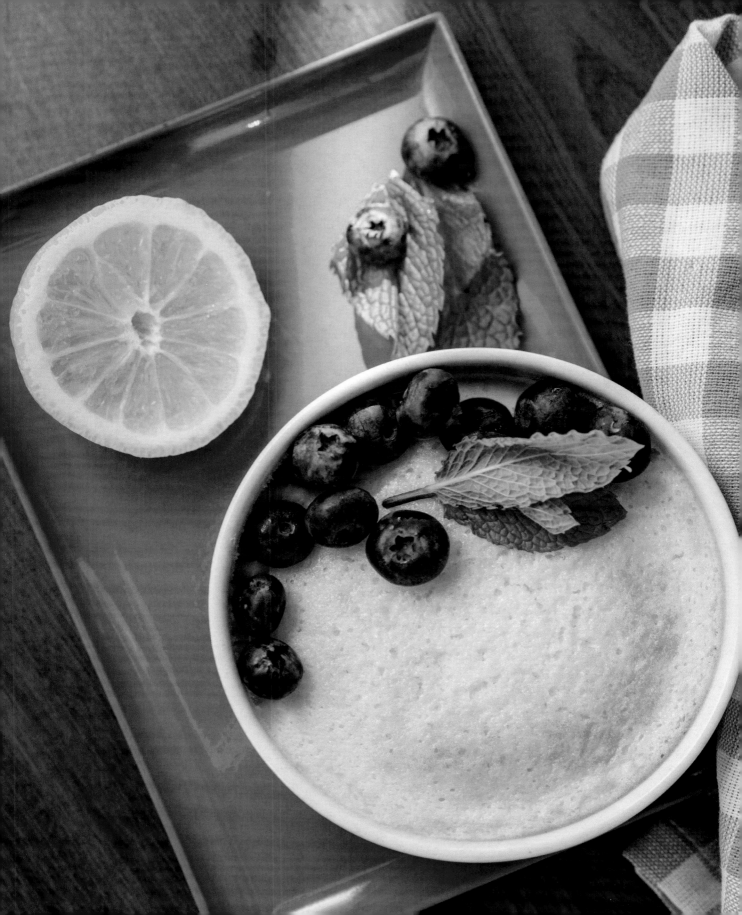

Vanilla bean panna cotta

SERVINGS: 6 | ●●

This quick, simple dessert is great year-round, but especially in the summer with fresh local berries added. Panna cotta is typically made with heavy cream. This version cuts down on the fat by using half-and-half. You can also replace 1 cup of the half-and-half with fat-free yogurt or Greek yogurt. If using yogurt, make sure to blend the mixture once it has cooled a little to intermix the yogurt with the hot liquid.

SHOPPING LIST: Half-and-half, vanilla bean, gelatin

CHECK FOR: Sugar

NUTRITIONAL ANALYSIS PER SERVING (1 RAMEKIN OR CUP MOLD): 130 calories, 6 g fat, 4 g saturated fat, 5 g protein, 17 g carbohydrates, 60 mg sodium

1 package gelatin
2 tablespoons cold water
3 cups half-and-half
½ cup sugar
1 vanilla bean, split open and scraped

Dissolve the gelatin packet in the cold water.

In a medium saucepan, add the half-and-half, sugar and vanilla bean. Bring the mixture to a boil.

Once the half-and-half mixture is boiling, whisk the dissolved gelatin into the hot liquid. If the gelatin has set already, that's fine. It should still dissolve into the hot liquid.

For single servings, pour the mixture into six ramekins or silicone cup molds and chill. You can also use an 8x8-inch cake pan and cut into squares to serve once it has solidified and chilled.

Fudgy brownies

SERVINGS: 12 |

To reduce the calories per serving, you can cut the brownies into smaller portions.

SHOPPING LIST: Unsweetened cocoa powder, low-fat vanilla yogurt, semisweet mini chocolate chips

CHECK FOR: Sugar, all-purpose flour, baking powder, salt, unsalted butter, eggs, vanilla, cooking spray

NUTRITIONAL ANALYSIS PER SERVING (1 PIECE): 130 calories, 4 g fat, 2.5 g saturated fat, 2 g protein, 24 g carbohydrates, 2 g fiber, 55 mg sodium

1 cup sugar
¾ cup all-purpose flour
⅓ cup unsweetened cocoa powder
½ teaspoon baking powder
¼ teaspoon salt
2 tablespoons unsalted butter
2 tablespoons low-fat vanilla yogurt
1 egg
2 teaspoons vanilla extract
¼ cup semi-sweet mini chocolate chips

Preheat oven to 350 F and lightly coat an 8x8-inch pan with cooking spray.

In a medium bowl, combine the sugar, flour, cocoa powder, baking powder and salt. Set aside.

Place the butter in a small saucepan and melt at medium-high heat. In a small bowl, combine the yogurt, egg and vanilla. Add the melted butter and mix.

Add the wet ingredients to the dry ingredients and mix well. The brownie batter will be stiff. Pour the batter into the prepared pan. Top with the chocolate chips.

Bake 15-20 minutes or until the brownies slightly puff up. Let cool and cut into 12 pieces.

Cranberry apple crisp

SERVINGS: 18 |

The filling for this crisp can be slowly cooked down and served as a topping (compote) for pancakes or light ice cream.

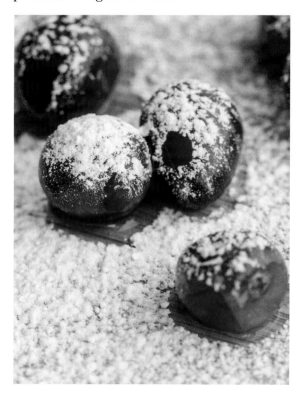

SHOPPING LIST: Granny Smith apples, cranberries, rolled oats, ground flax

CHECK FOR: Sugar, all-purpose flour, cinnamon, unsalted butter, brown sugar, cooking spray

NUTRITIONAL ANALYSIS PER SERVING (½ CUP): 140 calories, 4.5 g fat, 2 g saturated fat, 2 g protein, 25 g carbohydrates, 3 g fiber

6 cups Granny Smith apples, peeled and sliced
2 cups fresh or frozen cranberries
⅔ cup sugar
3 tablespoons all-purpose flour
½ teaspoon cinnamon

TOPPING
4 tablespoons unsalted butter, softened
¾ cup all-purpose flour
1 cup rolled oats
½ cup ground flax
⅓ cup brown sugar
½ teaspoon cinnamon

Preheat oven to 350 F. Lightly grease a 9x13-inch baking pan with cooking spray. (You can also use an oven-safe pot, as shown.)

Place apples, cranberries, sugar, flour and cinnamon in a bowl and toss until evenly coated. Spread the apple and cranberry mixture on the bottom of the pan.

Mix the softened butter, flour, oats, flax, brown sugar and cinnamon in bowl until butter is well incorporated into the flour mixture, forming crumbles.

Place the crumble mixture over the apples and cranberries. Bake 35-40 minutes.

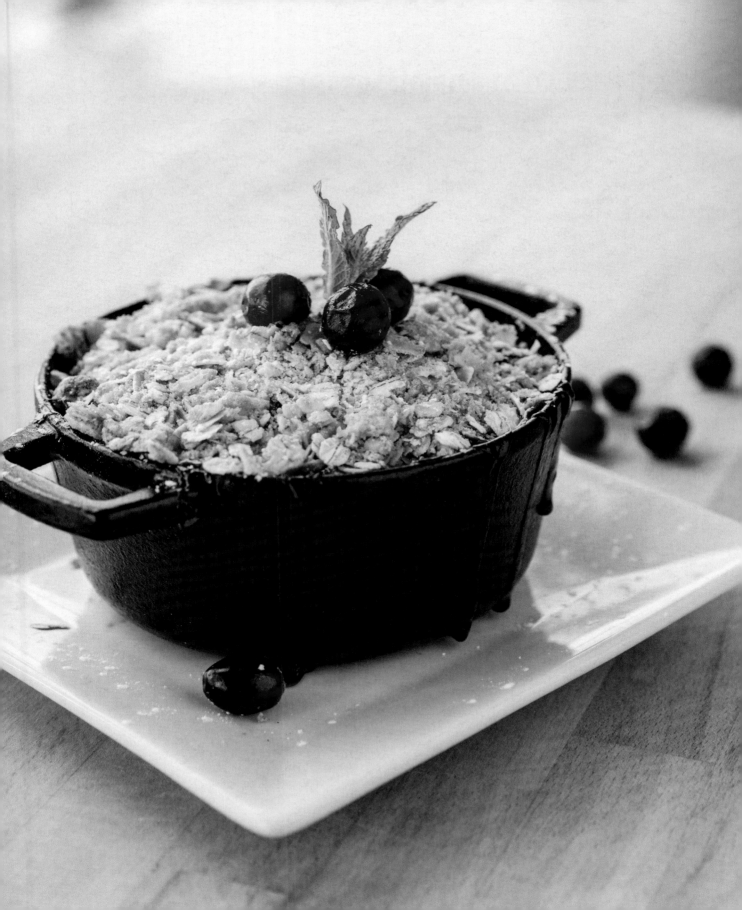

Spiced carrot cake

SERVINGS: 12 | ● ◖ ● ●

If you'd prefer to add some icing similar to typical carrot cake, beat together 8 ounces reduced-fat cream cheese, ½ cup powdered sugar and 1 teaspoon vanilla. You also can bake this cake in a cast-iron skillet for a different presentation and shape.

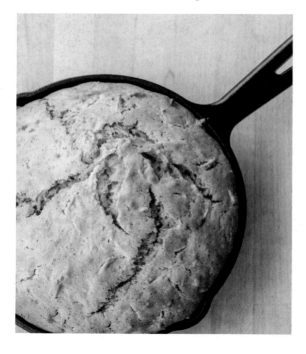

SHOPPING LIST: Fat-free plain yogurt, carrots

CHECK FOR: Sugar, canola oil, eggs, all-purpose flour, baking powder, baking soda, cinnamon, cloves, nutmeg, kosher salt, vanilla, cooking spray

NUTRITIONAL ANALYSIS PER SERVING (1 SLICE): 200 calories, 6 g fat, 1 g saturated fat, 6 g protein, 31 g carbohydrates, 1 g fiber, 330 mg sodium

1 cup sugar
¼ cup canola oil
1 cup fat-free plain yogurt
4 large eggs
2 cups all-purpose flour
2 teaspoons baking powder
2 teaspoons baking soda
2 teaspoons cinnamon
½ teaspoon cloves
¼ teaspoon nutmeg
½ teaspoon kosher salt
1 tablespoon vanilla extract
3 cups shredded carrots

Preheat oven to 350 F. Lightly grease two 8x8-inch cake pans with cooking spray.

In a large mixing bowl, add the sugar, yogurt, oil and eggs. Using an electric mixer, mix approximately 2-3 minutes to dissolve the sugar.

Add the dry ingredients and the vanilla and mix on medium speed about 1 minute until well incorporated. Fold or mix in the shredded carrots.

Divide the batter between the cake pans. Bake approximately 25 minutes, until a toothpick comes out clean in the center or the top of the cake bounces back when touched.

Slice each cake into 6 pieces. If desired, drizzle with a light cream cheese icing. Or cut each cake in half, placing one half on top of the other with a layer of icing between.

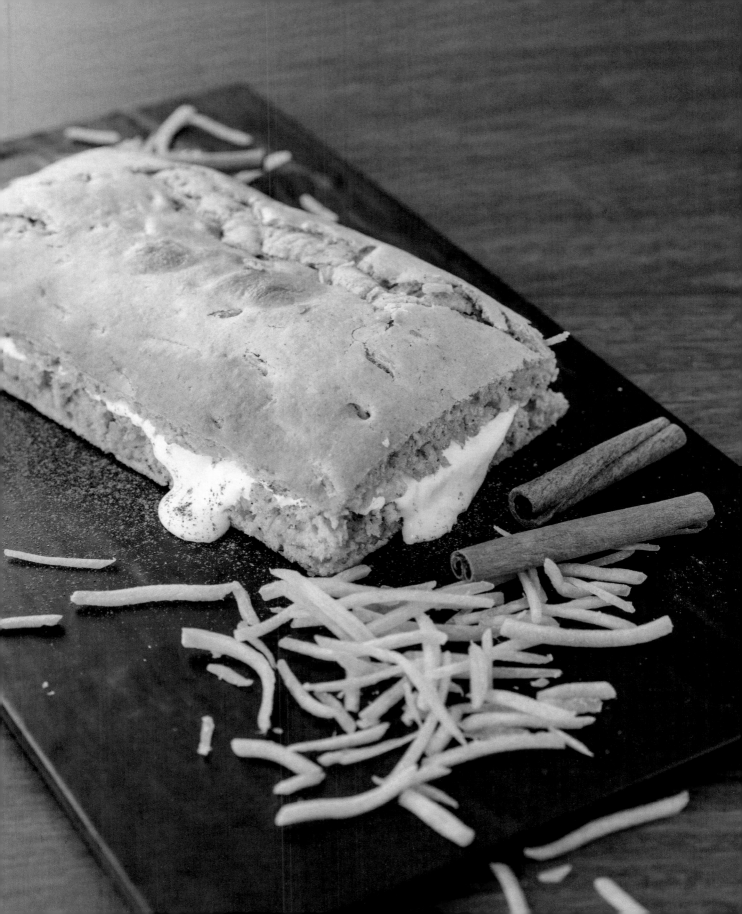

Chocolate soufflé

SERVINGS: 6 |

This dessert can be prepared 30 minutes before baking. Try not to open the oven door frequently to check on the progress of the desserts because they're very delicate. Serve hot.

3 ounces bittersweet chocolate (60%-70% cacao)
2 tablespoons + ¼ cup sugar, separated
1 egg yolk
¼ cup skim milk, brought to room temperature
2 egg whites, brought to room temperature
¼ teaspoon salt

AMARETTO CREAM (OPTIONAL)
1 cup fat-free Cool Whip or whipped topping
1 tablespoon amaretto liqueur

Preheat oven to 400 F. Spray six ramekins with cooking spray and sprinkle with 1 tablespoon of sugar.

Place chocolate in a heatproof bowl. Microwave 30 seconds at a time, stirring every 30 seconds until melted, or place the bowl over a pot of boiling water and stir frequently.

Add the ¼ cup sugar and the egg yolk and stir until blended well. Remove from heat, and stir in milk. Set aside and let cool.

Place the egg whites and salt in a small bowl. Using an electric mixer at medium-high speed, beat the egg whites until soft peaks form. Add the remaining tablespoon of sugar and beat on high speed until stiff peaks form.

Place ¼ of the egg white mixture in the chocolate mixture and combine. Slowly add the chocolate mixture to the egg white mixture, small amounts at a time, gently folding with a rubber spatula. DO NOT STIR. You don't want to lose the air that's mixed in.

Place ⅓ cup of chocolate soufflé mixture in each ramekin. Bake 15-20 minutes, or until tops are lightly golden.

While the soufflés are baking, combine the Cool Whip and amaretto. Place a small spoonful of the topping on each soufflé when ready to eat, as the topping will melt quickly.

SHOPPING LIST: Bittersweet chocolate, Cool Whip (optional), amaretto liqueur (optional)

CHECK FOR: Sugar, eggs, skim milk, salt, cooking spray

NUTRITIONAL ANALYSIS PER SERVING (1 SOUFFLÉ): 140 calories, 7 g fat, 3.5 g saturated fat, 3 g protein, 17 g carbohydrates, 2 g fiber, 65 mg sodium

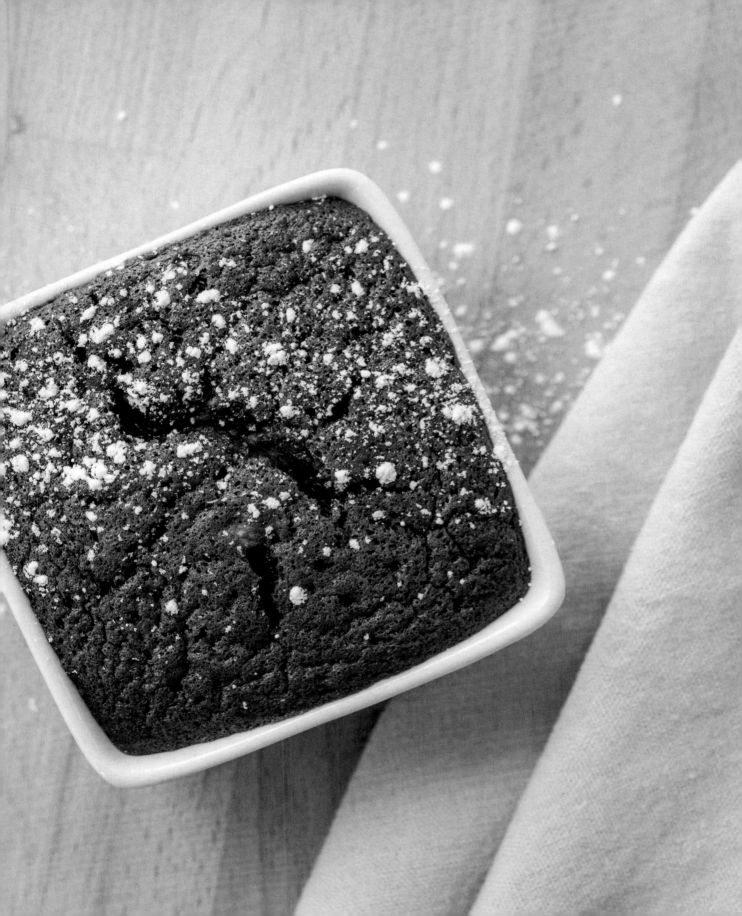

Pumpkin spice soufflé

SERVINGS: 8 |

The most important part of a soufflé is to make sure you handle it with care and serve it immediately out of the oven, as it will lose its height relatively quickly. If your timing is off, you can always call your soufflé a "fallen soufflé" — the taste will be the same.

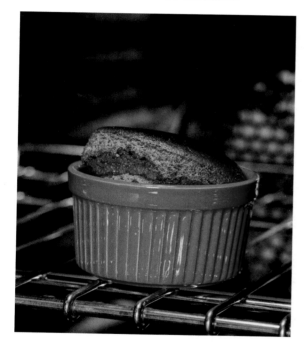

1 tablespoon sugar
1 cup skim milk
2 tablespoons cornstarch
1 cup pumpkin purée
½ teaspoon cinnamon
¼ teaspoon ground nutmeg
¼ teaspoon ground cloves
¾ cup sugar
¼ teaspoon salt
10 egg whites

Preheat oven to 400 F. Lightly spray eight 6-ounce ramekins with cooking spray. Sprinkle the ramekins with the tablespoon of sugar and place on a baking sheet.

In a medium sauté pan, add the skim milk, cornstarch, pumpkin purée, cinnamon, nutmeg and cloves. Then add ¼ cup of the sugar. Turn the heat to medium high, and stir continuously until the mixture comes to a boil and starts to thicken. Remove from heat and let cool.

In a separate bowl, whip the egg whites about 2 minutes with an electric mixer, adding the salt, until stiff peaks form. Slowly add the remaining ½ cup of sugar and whip an additional minute until the eggs are stiff and glossy.

Taste the cooled pumpkin mixture to make sure the flavor is strong; add more spices if desired. Gently fold the mixture in with the egg whites. Place equal portions into the ramekins. Reduce the oven to 375 F and bake about 20 minutes, or until the center is firm and slightly golden brown. Serve immediately.

SHOPPING LIST: Pumpkin purée

CHECK FOR: Sugar, cornstarch, skim milk, cinnamon, nutmeg, cloves, salt, eggs, cooking spray

NUTRITIONAL ANALYSIS PER SERVING (1 SOUFFLÉ): 100 calories, 6 g protein, 21 g carbohydrates, 1 g fiber, 140 mg sodium

Angel food cake

Angel food cake is a slightly delicate dessert to make, but don't be intimidated. Practice makes perfect. Still, even imperfect angel food cake rarely disappoints!

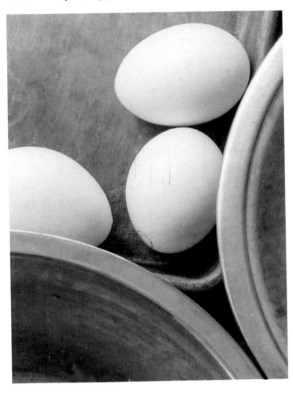

SHOPPING LIST: Lemon

CHECK FOR: Eggs, cream of tartar, salt, sugar, cake flour, vanilla

NUTRITIONAL ANALYSIS PER SERVING (1 SLICE OR CUPCAKE): 120 calories, 5 g protein, 27 g carbohydrates, 95 mg sodium

12 large egg whites, room temperature
1 teaspoon cream of tartar
¼ teaspoon salt
1 ½ cup sugar
1 cup cake flour
1 teaspoon vanilla extract
1 teaspoon lemon zest (using 1 whole lemon)

Preheat oven to 350 F.

Place the egg whites in large mixing bowl. Make sure they're at room temperature as they'll whip much better than if they're cold.

With an electric mixer, using the whisk attachment if you have one, beat the egg whites on medium-high speed about 1-2 minutes.

Add the cream of tartar and salt and mix an additional 2-3 minutes. Gradually add the sugar until the egg whites form stiff peaks.

Sift in the cake flour and add the vanilla extract and lemon zest. Carefully fold these ingredients into the egg whites.

Pour the mixture into an ungreased 10-inch angel food cake (tube) pan, or you can prepare the mixture as 12 cupcakes. Bake 35-40 minutes. The bake time will be less if you're making cupcakes.

Zucchini bread

The fat-free plain Greek yogurt in this recipe helps reduce the amount of oil needed. It also helps increase the protein content of the zucchini bread and keep it moist. For a simple flavor variation, try shredded carrots in place of the shredded zucchini and add ½ teaspoon of ground cloves.

SHOPPING LIST: Ground flaxseed, fat-free plain Greek yogurt, zucchini

CHECK FOR: All-purpose flour, sugar, baking soda, baking powder, cinnamon, eggs, canola oil, vanilla, cooking spray

NUTRITIONAL ANALYSIS PER SERVING (1 SLICE): 150 calories, 7 g fat, 0.5 g saturated fat, 3 g protein, 19 g carbohydrates, 2 g fiber, 65 mg sodium

1 cup ground flaxseed
2 cups all-purpose flour
1 ½ cups sugar
1 teaspoon baking soda
1 teaspoon baking powder
1 tablespoon cinnamon
3 large eggs
½ cup canola oil
½ cup fat-free plain Greek yogurt
1 tablespoon vanilla extract
2 cups shredded zucchini

Preheat the oven to 350 F.

If you have an electric mixer, place all of the dry ingredients in a mixing bowl and combine, using a paddle attachment if you have one. Add the eggs, oil, yogurt and vanilla and mix until well incorporated. Fold in the zucchini.

If you don't have an electric mixer, combine the dry ingredients in a mixing bowl and create a well in the middle. Add the wet ingredients to the well, and whisk together by hand until blended well. Fold in the zucchini.

Spray two loaf pans with cooking spray. Divide the batter between the two and bake approximately 45 minutes, or until a tooth-pick placed in the middle of the bread comes out clean.

Let the bread cool in the pan 2-3 minutes. Then flip the bread on its side to help release it from the pan and let it cool more efficiently. Slice each loaf into 12 pieces. Bread slices better after cooling at least 15 minutes. Freeze what you won't be eating during the week.

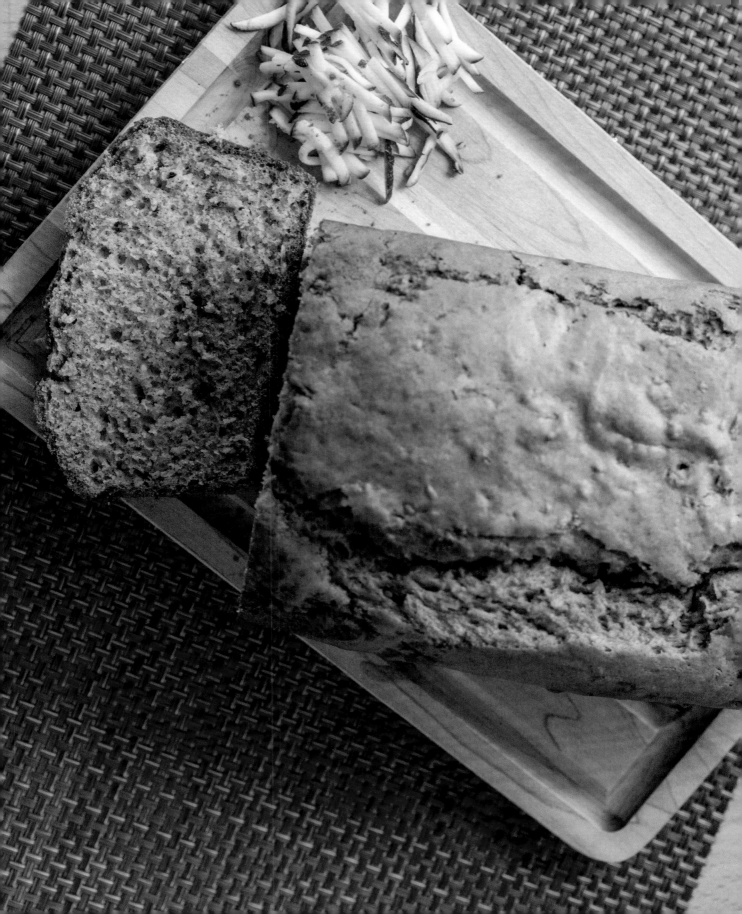

Apple cider compote

SERVINGS: 4 |

Compotes make great toppings. Serve over French toast, pancakes, whole-grain waffles, or on oatmeal.

SHOPPING LIST: Granny Smith apples, apple juice or cider

CHECK FOR: Brown sugar, cinnamon, cornstarch (optional)

NUTRITIONAL ANALYSIS PER SERVING: (½ CUP): 98 calories, 25 g carbohydrates, 6 mg sodium

2 Granny Smith apples, peeled, cored and sliced
1 ½ cup apple juice or cider
1 tablespoon brown sugar
½ teaspoon ground cinnamon
2 teaspoons cornstarch + 2 teaspoons cold water (optional)

Warm a saucepan over medium heat. Add the apple slices and cook approximately 5 minutes, stirring frequently.

Add the apple juice or cider, brown sugar, and cinnamon. Bring the mixture to a simmer, stirring frequently until the apples are tender and the sauce has a slight thickness to it.

If a thicker sauce is desired, add small amounts of cornstarch mixed with cold water until the sauce reaches the desired consistency. The compote will continue to thicken as it cools.

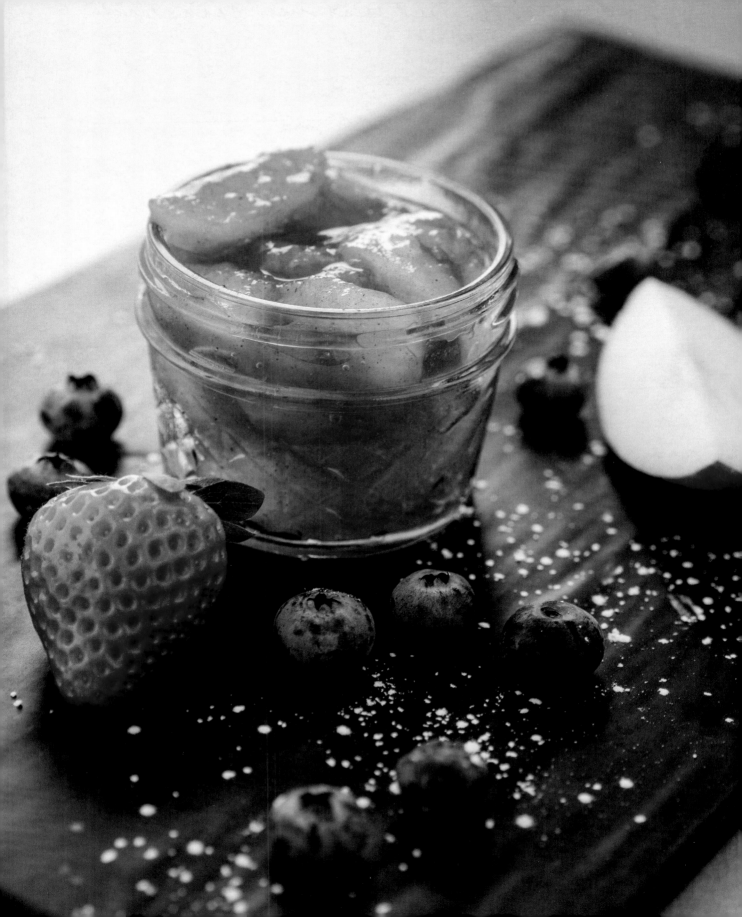

★★★★★ great! Did not use cornstarch. Very good!!

Strawberry compote

SERVINGS: 4 | ◖◗

If you have strawberries in your fridge that are slightly past their prime or becoming weathered, this compote is a great way to put them to use and enjoy their flavor. Making a compote is a good trick for using up other types of bruised or imperfect fruits, as long as they're not rotting.

SHOPPING LIST: Strawberries

CHECK FOR: Sugar, cornstarch (optional)

NUTRITIONAL ANALYSIS PER SERVING
(¼ CUP): 30 calories, 1 g protein, 3 g carbohydrates

2 cups cleaned and quartered strawberries
1 tablespoon sugar
2 teaspoons cornstarch + 2 teaspoons cold water (optional)

Warm a saucepan over medium heat. Add the strawberries and cook approximately 5 minutes, stirring frequently.

Add the sugar. Keep stirring frequently while bringing the mixture to a simmer. Cook until the strawberries are tender and the sauce has a slight thickness to it.

If a thicker sauce is desired, add small amounts of cornstarch mixed with cold water until the sauce reaches the desired consistency. The compote will continue to thicken as it cools.

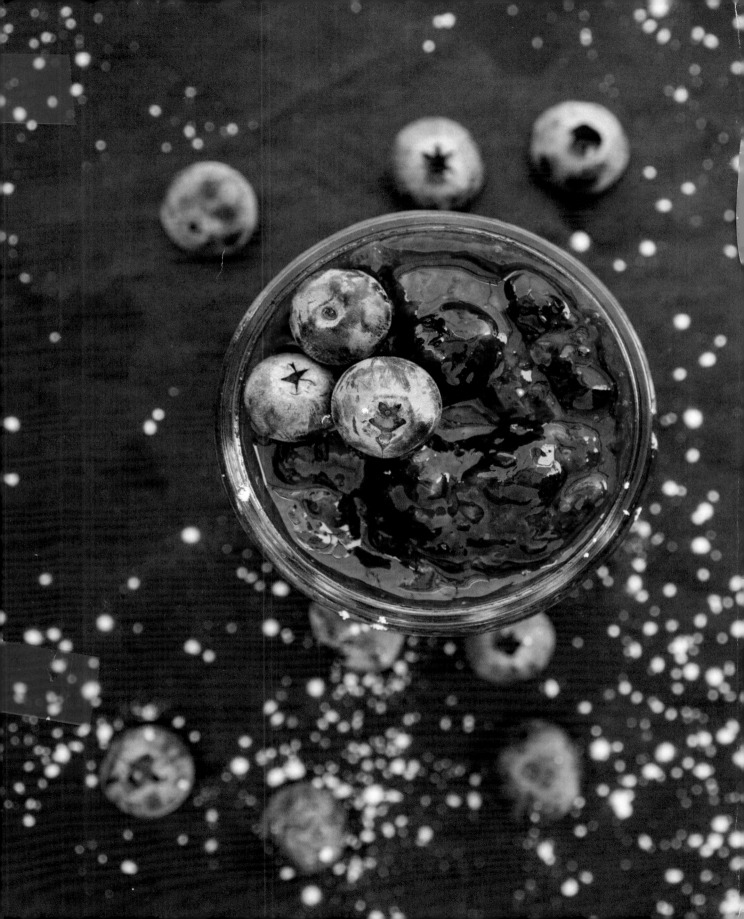

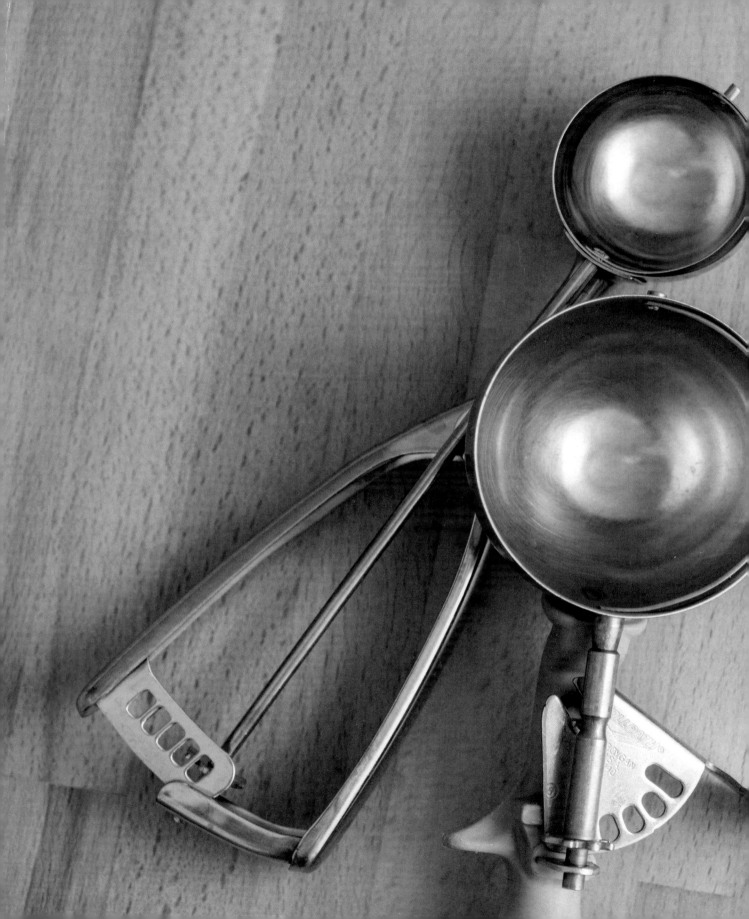

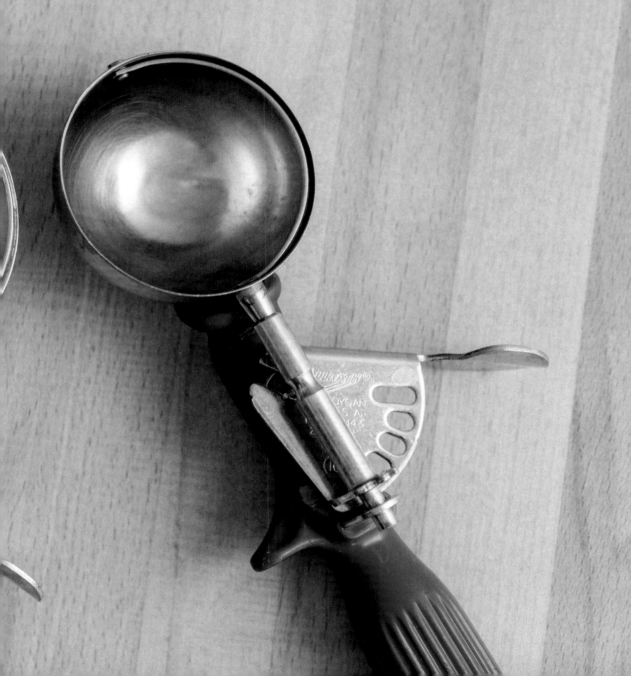

Appendix

Cooking glossary

AL DENTE | To cook something, often pasta or rice, leaving it with a bit of firmness.

BAKE | To cook food in an oven using dry heat.

BASTE | To moisten food and add flavor by spooning, bushing or squirting liquid on the food while it cooks.

BEAT | To stir rapidly in a circular motion with a whisk, spoon or mixer.

BLACKEN | To season generously and cook over high heat in a heavy, very hot skillet until the food item is charred, creating a crispy, spicy crust (a Cajun style of cooking).

BLANCHE | To create a crisp-tender texture and keep colors bright by placing vegetables in boiling water for 1-5 minutes and then placing them in cold water to stop the cooking process.

BLEND | To thoroughly combine two or more ingredients with a whisk, spoon or mixer.

BOIL | To cook food in a liquid at a high temperature (at least 212 F) that causes bubbles to form in the liquid.

BREAD | To coat with breadcrumbs, crackers or flour.

BROIL | To cook under direct high heat, usually in an oven or a broiler.

BROWN | To cook over high heat for a short period, on all sides, giving the food a brown appearance.

BUTTERFLY | To split through the center to open and thin out.

CARAMELIZE | To heat sugar until it liquefies and becomes a brown syrup, or to break down the natural sugars in vegetables, such as onions, bell peppers and carrots.

CHOP | To cut into small, slightly irregular cubes or pieces.

CORE | To remove the seeds or the tough woody centers of fruits and vegetables.

CUBE | To cut food into small (about ½-inch) cubes.

DASH | To add a small amount of an ingredient, roughly ⅛ teaspoon.

DEGLAZE | To loosen brown bits from a pan by adding liquid, and then heating the liquid while scraping the pan.

DICE | To cut into very small cubes (about ⅛- to ¼-inch).

DILUTE | To reduce the strength of a mixture by adding liquid.

DREDGE | To cover or coat uncooked food, usually with flour, cornmeal or breadcrumbs.

DUST | To coat lightly with powdered (confectioners') sugar, cocoa or another powdery ingredient.

EMULSIFY | To combine liquids or semi-liquids that don't naturally mix together.

FILLET | To cut away the bones from a piece of meat, poultry or fish, or in reference to a flat piece of boneless meat.

FLORET | To break or cut fresh broccoli or cauliflower into small clusters.

FRY | To cook food in a hot oil over medium to high heat until brown and crisp.

GARNISH | To decorate a finished food with an herb, fruit or vegetable.

GRATE | To rub foods against a serrated surface to produce fine, shredded bits.

GREASE | To rub the interior surface of a cooking dish or pan with shortening, butter or cooking spray to prevent food from sticking.

GRILL | To cook food on a rack over direct heat, such as on a barbecue grill or a smoke-less indoor grill, or to cook food in a cast iron skillet placed on an outdoor grill rack.

JULIENNE | To cut in a shape that resembles matchsticks.

KNEAD | To work dough by hand or in a mixer with a dough hook until it forms into a smooth ball.

MARINATE | To soak in a flavored liquid before cooking or preparation.

MINCE | To cut into tiny pieces.

PARBOIL | To partially cook food by boiling it, usually to prepare the food for final cooking using another method.

PINCH | To add a tiny amount of an ingredient, literally the amount of spice you can pinch between your fingers.

POACH | To cook over low heat in liquid that's barely simmering and just covers the food.

PURÉE | To mash or grind food until completely smooth, usually in a food processor or blender.

REDUCE | To lessen the amount of liquid and strengthen its favor by simmering it slowly.

ROAST | To cook a large piece of meat or poultry uncovered in an oven using dry heat.

SAUTÉ | To cook food in a small amount of oil or shortening over relatively high heat.

SCALD | To heat liquid almost to a boil, until small bubbles begin to form on the edges.

SEAR | To cook meat over very high heat for a short period in order to seal in the meat's juices.

SHRED | To cut into fine strips with a grater.

SIFT | To pass a small amount of an ingredient, such as flour or powdered sugar, through a sieve or sifter to make it smooth.

SIMMER | To cook in a liquid just below the boiling point so that bubbles form but they don't burst on the surface.

SKIM | To spoon off the top layer of foam, fat or impurities floating to the top.

SLICE | To cut food into thin, flat pieces.

STEAM | To cook over boiling water using a covered kettle or metal basket with holes in the bottom (steamer).

STIR-FRY | To quickly cook small pieces of food over high heat, stirring constantly.

WHISK | To beat the ingredients by hand using a whisk or fork to incorporate air into the mixture.

ZEST | To remove the outer portion of a citrus fruit peel by scraping it into fine pieces.

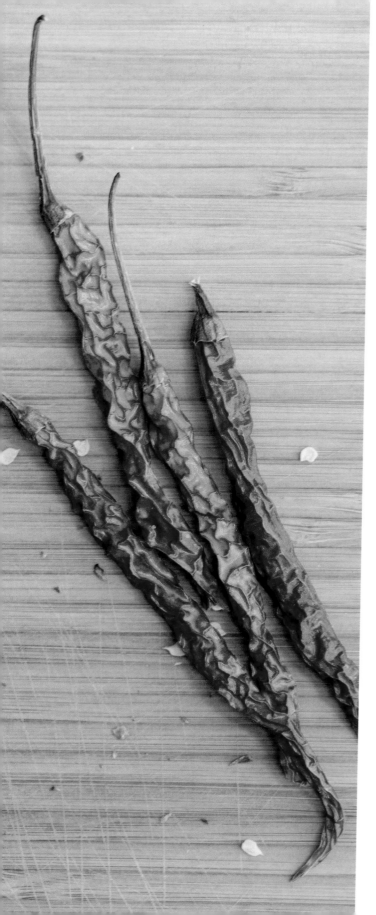

Herbs and spices

Food is all about flavor, and a great way to enhance the flavor of foods is with herbs and spices. Adding herbs and spices while cooking brings out the natural flavor of meat and turns ordinary vegetables, soups and side dishes into tasty accompaniments.

Herbs originate from the fresh part of a plant — the leaves, flowers and stems. A spice comes from the dried part of a plant — its roots, bark, seeds or dried fruits.

The chart on the opposite page describes some common herbs and spices used in cooking. Below are basic herb and spice rubs that you can make in advance to flavor your meats, seafood and even vegetables.

Barbecue rub
½ cup paprika
½ cup brown sugar
2 tablespoons ground black pepper
2 tablespoons salt
2 teaspoons dry mustard
2 teaspoons cayenne pepper

Italian herb rub
2 tablespoons dried basil
2 tablespoons dried oregano
1 tablespoon garlic powder
1 tablespoon onion powder
1 teaspoon ground fennel
1 teaspoon salt
¼ teaspoon pepper

Souvlaki rub
2 tablespoons olive oil
1 tablespoon minced garlic
1 tablespoon fresh oregano
1 teaspoon salt
½ teaspoon ground black pepper

	FLAVOR	IS IT SPICY?	GOES WELL WITH	SUGGESTED AMOUNT
BASIL	Warm, savory and a little sweet, with hints of peppery tones	No	Fresh vegetables, breading mixtures, poultry, meat, fish, Italian dishes	If using fresh, it's always three times the amount of dried.
CAYENNE	Hot and fiery with a strong bite	Yes	Chili, egg bakes, chicken, meat, fish, tofu, soups	¼ teaspoon
CHILI POWDER	Fruity and smoky to superhot, depending on the pepper	Yes	Chili, soups, sauces, stews, poultry, meat, fish, seasoning blends	1 teaspoon
CINNAMON	Woody and sweet	No	Breads, cakes, oatmeal, beverages, fruits, jams, chicken, Middle Eastern dishes	½-1 teaspoon
CUMIN	Both sweet and bitter with a warm and earthy aroma	No	Beans, lentils, soups, stews, tacos, vegetables, Moroccan dishes	1 teaspoon
GARLIC	Pungent and slightly bitter in raw form, mild and sweet when sautéed	No	Most cuisines, salsas, spreads, sauces, oils, meat, fish, vegetables	1 teaspoon–1 tablespoon
GINGER	Slightly peppery and sweet with a pungent and refreshing aroma	No	Stir-fry, poultry, beef, vegetables, sauces, desserts, Thai dishes	1 teaspoon–1 tablespoon
OREGANO	Bold and earthy with a slight bitterness	No	Pizza, sauces, pasta, rubs, soups, vegetables, Mexican and Mediterranean dishes	1 teaspoon
PAPRIKA	Bitter with a hint of smoke and sweetness	No	Rubs, chili, soups, sauces, legumes, vegetables, potatoes	1 teaspoon
RED PEPPER FLAKES	Sharp and biting with mild heat, adding warmth to the tongue	Yes	Chili, sauces, rubs, dressings, meats, seafood, South American and Asian dishes	¼ teaspoon

Making conversions

It's not uncommon when cooking or baking that you need to make some conversions. Maybe you cut the recipe in half and now you're not sure exactly how much of a certain ingredient you need. Or perhaps you purchased an ingredient in bulk and you need to determine how much is equivalent to 4 ounces.

Making conversions can sometimes be confusing, especially if you don't do it often. The information below can help simplify common cooking conversions.

Keep in mind when shredding items, such as cheese, that shredding basically doubles the volume. So, if a recipe calls for 1 cup of shredded cheese and you're shredding the cheese, you'll want to shred about 4 ounces of cheese (not 8 ounces).

On the chart below, the measurements within each row are equivalents. For example, 4 tablespoons equals ¼ cup or 2 ounces or 60 milliliters or ⅛ pound.

3 teaspoons	1 tablespoon	½ ounce	15 milliliters	
2 tablespoons	⅛ cup	1 ounce	30 milliliters	
4 tablespoons	¼ cup	2 ounces	60 milliliters	⅛ pound
8 tablespoons	½ cup	4 ounces	125 milliliters	¼ pound
16 tablespoons	1 cup	8 ounces	250 milliliters	½ pound
1 pint	2 cups	16 ounces	.5 liters	1 pound
1 quart	4 cups	32 ounces	.95 liters	2 pounds
1 gallon	4 quarts	128 ounces	3.8 liters	8 ⅓ pounds

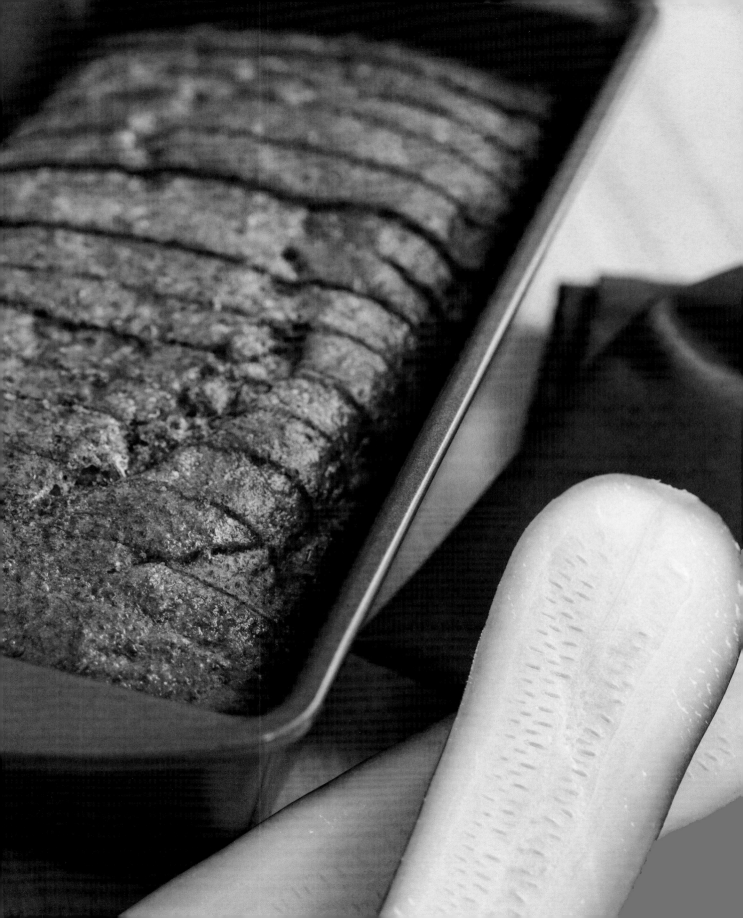

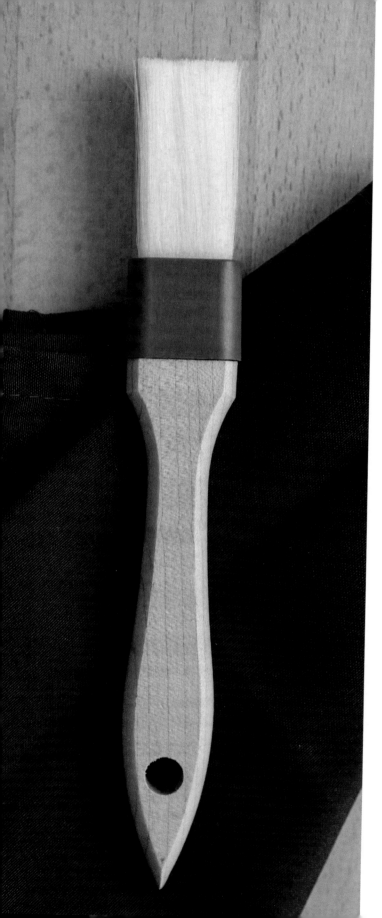

Adapting recipes

Your grandmother's beloved bread pudding is scrumptious, but it may not be healthy. That doesn't mean you can't enjoy her bread pudding and some of your other favorite recipes on occasion. And chances are, with some simple changes you can prepare your favorite foods with added nutrition and less fat and calories.

On the opposite page are techniques for transforming less healthy recipes into healthier ones — without losing out on taste. You can also use this information if you're out of a particular ingredient and you don't feel like going to the store to buy more.

Other techniques for making foods more nutritious are based on cooking technique. Can you cook the food item a different way? Roasting, baking or steaming foods, for example, is healthier than frying them in butter or shortening.

Cooking without gluten
If you want to take one of your favorite recipes and make it gluten-free, or your goal is to eat less gluten, here are some basic tips.

If the recipe calls for all-purpose flour, use a gluten-free flour instead. Common options include oat flour, almond flour and rice flour. They're available in most grocery stores. For oat flour, make sure it's made from certified gluten-free oats.

If the recipe uses flour as a thickening agent, substitute with cornstarch, arrowroot powder or tapioca flour instead.

If the recipe calls for breadcrumbs, purchase a gluten-free cereal and make your own breading with crushed cereal.

IF THE RECIPE CALLS FOR:	SUBSTITUTE WITH THE FOLLOWING:
BUTTER MARGARINE SHORTENING OIL	For baked goods, substitute half the butter, shortening or oil with pureed low-fat cottage cheese, mashed banana, prune or pumpkin purée, or fat-free yogurt. For stove-top cooking, sauté food in broth or small amounts of healthy oils such as olive, canola or peanut. (If using cooking spray, keep in mind that you'll have to keep the heat significantly lower.)
WHOLE MILK (REGULAR OR EVAPORATED)	Use fat-free or 1% milk, or evaporated skim milk.
CREAM	Use half-and-half.
A WHOLE EGG (YOLK AND WHITE)	Use ¼ cup egg substitute or 2 egg whites.
SOUR CREAM OR CREAM CHEESE	For dips, spreads, dressings and toppings, use low-fat or light varieties, non-fat Greek yogurt, or low-fat cottage cheese that's puréed in a blender or food processor. Fat-free, low-fat and light varieties may not work as well for baking.
CHEESE	In recipes that call for 1 cup of shredded cheese, the amount can often be reduced by half, especially if using a pungent cheese such as sharp cheddar, pepper jack, feta and aged Parmesan.
MAYONNAISE	Use non-fat Greek yogurt or light mayo.
SUGAR	In many baked goods, you can reduce the amount of sugar by one-third to one-half without affecting the texture or taste. But use no less than ¼ cup sugar for every cup of flour to keep items moist. To boost sweetness when reducing sugar, add spices such as cinnamon, cloves, nutmeg, or flavoring such as vanilla or almond. In place of sugar, use honey or sugar substitutes such as sucrose or sucralose.
WHITE FLOUR	Replace half of the white flour with whole-grain regular or pastry flour. Note: When substituting whole-wheat flour for white flour, you may need to add more moisture.
SALT	For baked goods, reduce the amount of salt by up to half. This does not apply to yeast-leavened items, such as bread. When cooking or frying, use herbs and spices. Add salt toward the end of food preparation if needed and use sparingly. Adding lime and lemon juice can enhance the salt flavor.
BREADCRUMBS	Use rolled oats or crushed cereal. If you need gluten-free, use Rice Krispies, Rice Squares, cornflakes or another gluten-free cereal.
WHITE RICE	Use brown rice, wild rice, bulgur wheat or pearl barley.
WHITE (ENRICHED) PASTA	Use whole-wheat pasta.
GROUND BEEF	Replace half the beef in casseroles, soups and stews with vegetables, red quinoa, ground turkey or chicken breast, lentils, or textured vegetable protein. Use leaner cuts of beef.

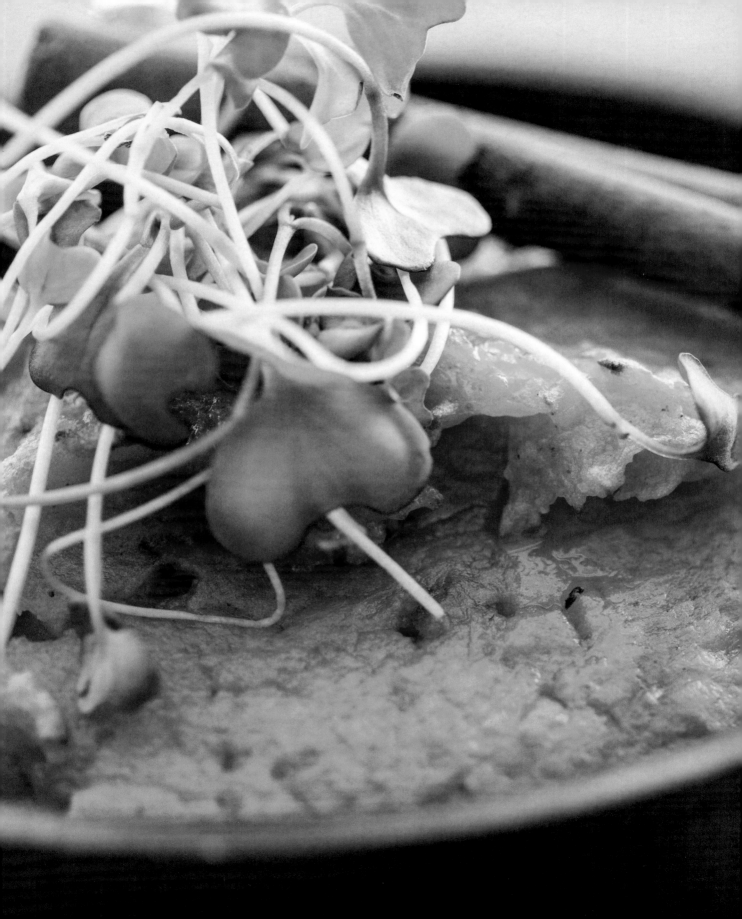

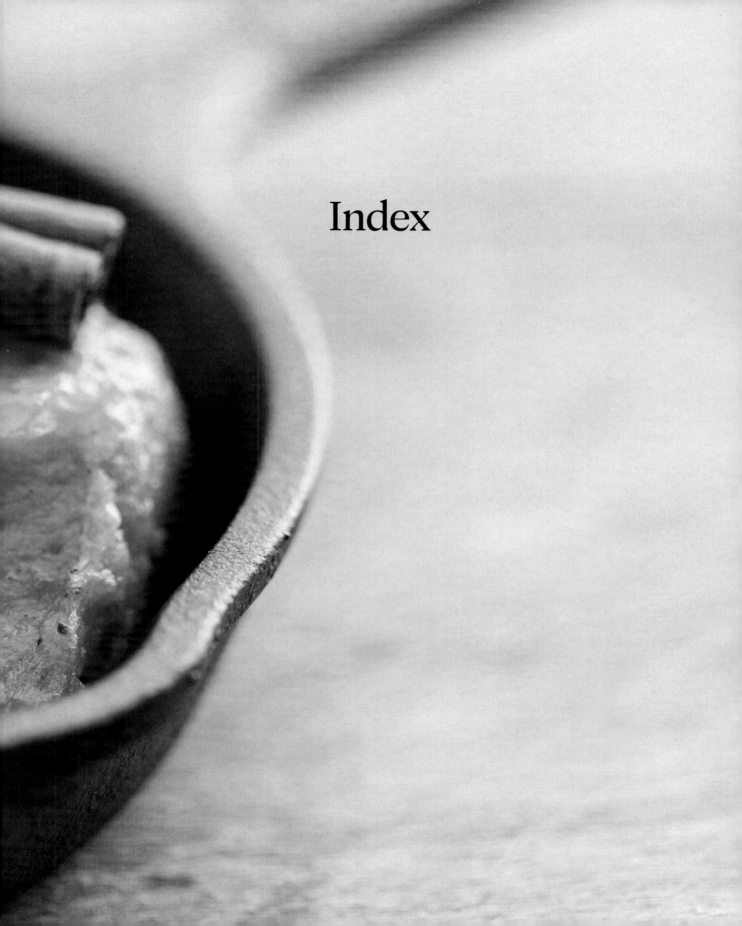

Index

A

appetizers and snacks
    basil pesto stuffed mushrooms, 108
    black bean and corn salsa, 98
    buffalo zucchini sticks, 110
    coconut shrimp, 104
    roasted red pepper hummus, 100
    spinach artichoke dip, 102
    Thai chicken satay, 106
    tomato bruschetta, 103
apples and cider
    apple cider compote, 244
    cranberry apple crisp, 234
    cranberry apple oatmeal, 65

B

baking, 28
baking sheets and pans, 17
banana flax pancakes, 46
barley risotto with vegetables, 138
basil
    basil pesto, 201
    pesto stuffed mushrooms, 108
    tomato, basil and mozzarella hoagie, 74
beans
    black bean and corn salsa, 98
    black bean burgers, 186
    black bean quesadillas, 188
    Cuban black bean soup, 84
    minestrone soup, 94
    roasted red pepper hummus, 100
    Southwest taco bowl, 182
    three bean chili, 95
    white bean and kale soup, 90
beef
    carne asada, 176
    hearty beef lasagna, 174
    Santa Fe lime fajitas, 157
    selecting, 21
    shepherd's pie, 180
    Swedish meatballs with quinoa, 178
    sweet and savory meatloaf, 171
    three bean chili, 95

beets, thyme-roasted, 120
bell peppers
    black bean and corn salsa, 98
    black bean quesadillas, 188
    breakfast potatoes, 52
    California avocado wrap, 68
    cutting, 24
    edamame pad thai, 190
    Greek pasta salad, 78
    Greek roasted vegetables, 128
    grilled vegetable kebabs, 126
    pita pizza, 222
    roasted red pepper hummus, 100
    roasted red pepper pineapple salsa, 158
    roasted sweet potato hash, 51
    romesco sauce, 205
    Santa Fe lime fajitas, 157
    Southwest taco bowl, 182
    vegetable lasagna roll-ups, 219
    vegetable stir-fry, 124
blueberry pancakes, 50
breading, 28
breakfast
    banana flax pancakes, 46
    blueberry pancakes, 50
    breakfast potatoes, 52
    broccoli and smoked Gouda frittata, 60
    caprese frittata, 62
    cheesy poached egg sandwich, 54
    chicken or turkey sausage patties, 56
    cinnamon carrot pancakes, 48
    cranberry apple oatmeal, 65
    orange cinnamon French toast, 58
    power morning muffins, 57
    roasted sweet potato hash, 51
    Southwest frittata, 64
    whole-wheat French toast, 59
broccoli
    broccoli and smoked Gouda frittata, 60
    broccoli cheddar soup, 88
    broccoli cheddar tofu cakes, 191
    broccoli macaroni bites, 224
broiling, 28
bruschetta, tomato, 103
Brussels sprouts, balsamic-glazed, 116
butternut squash fries, 114

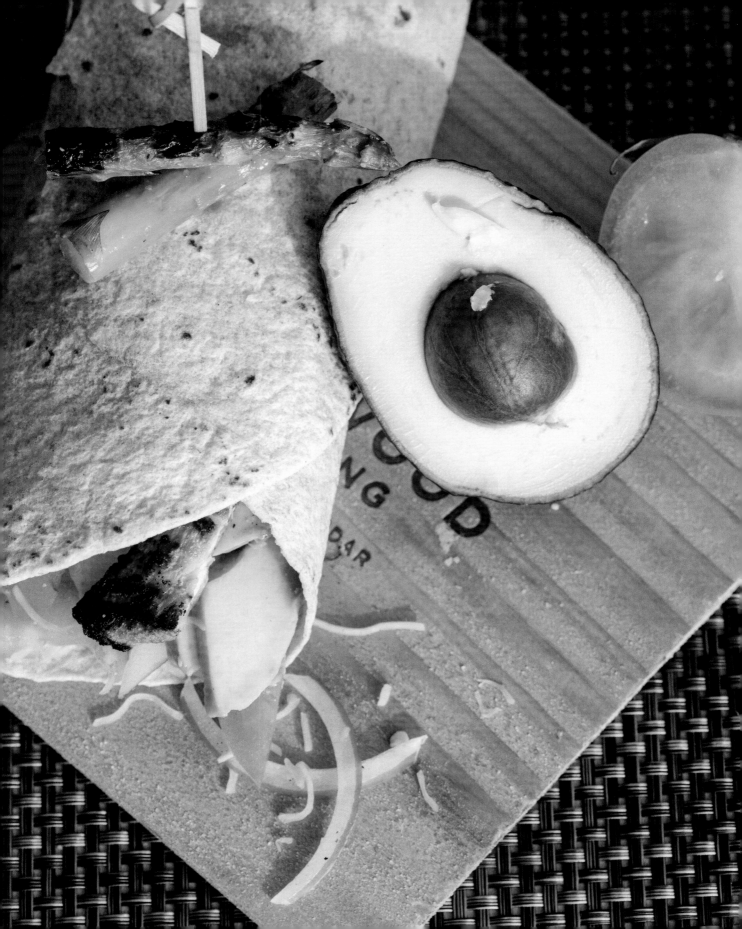

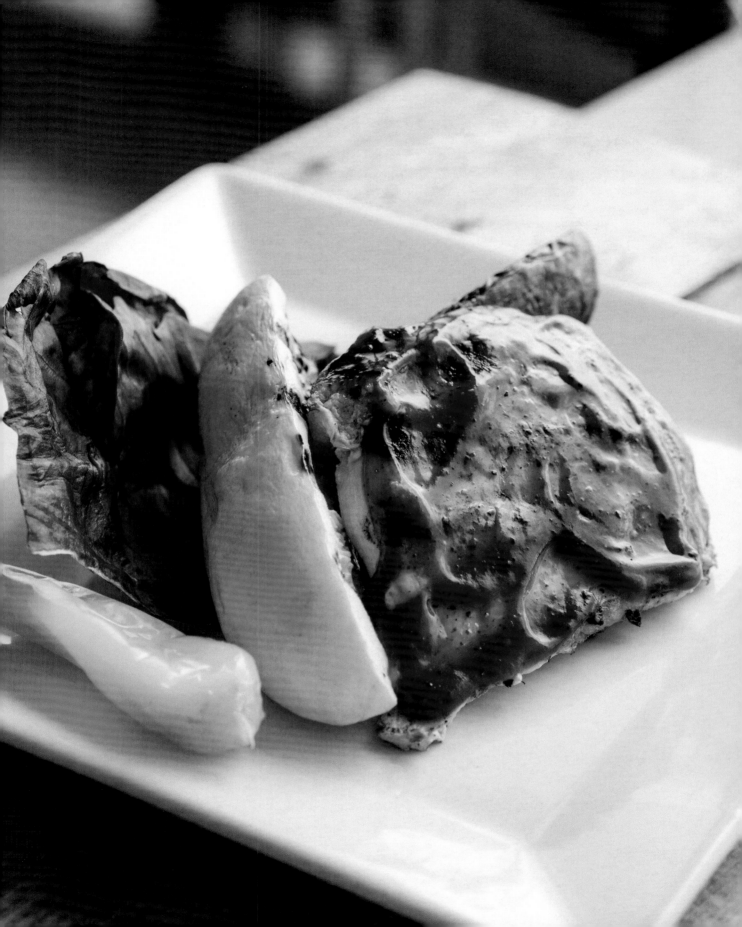

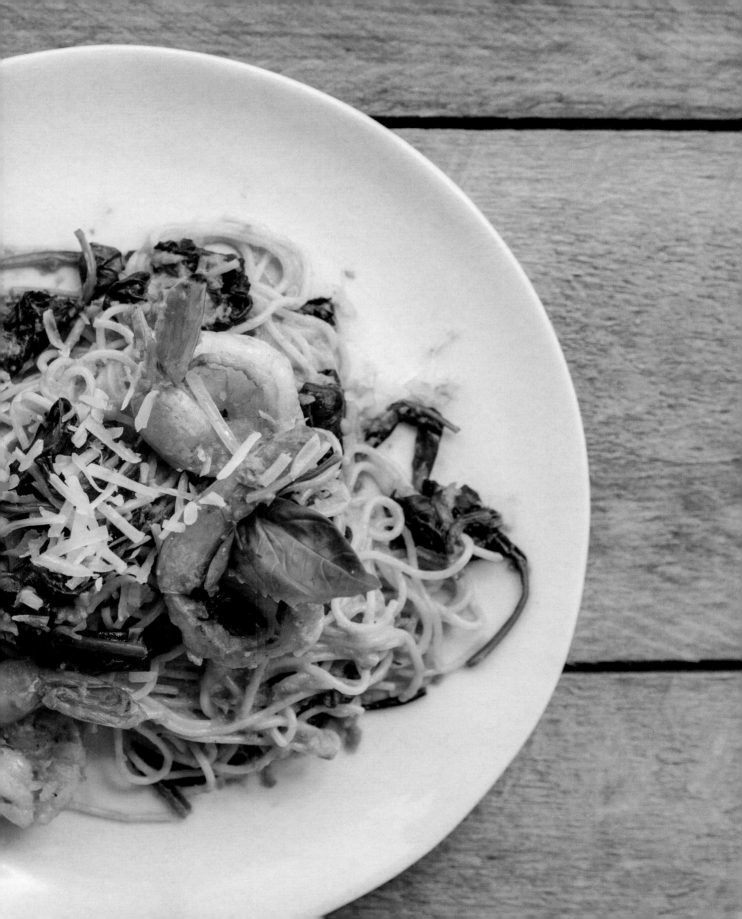

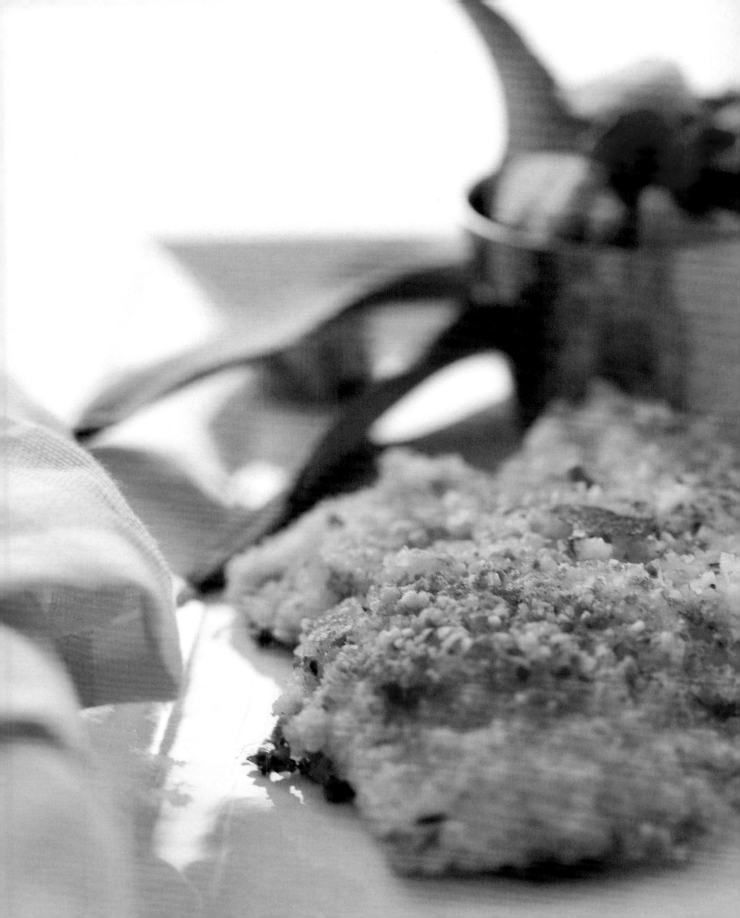

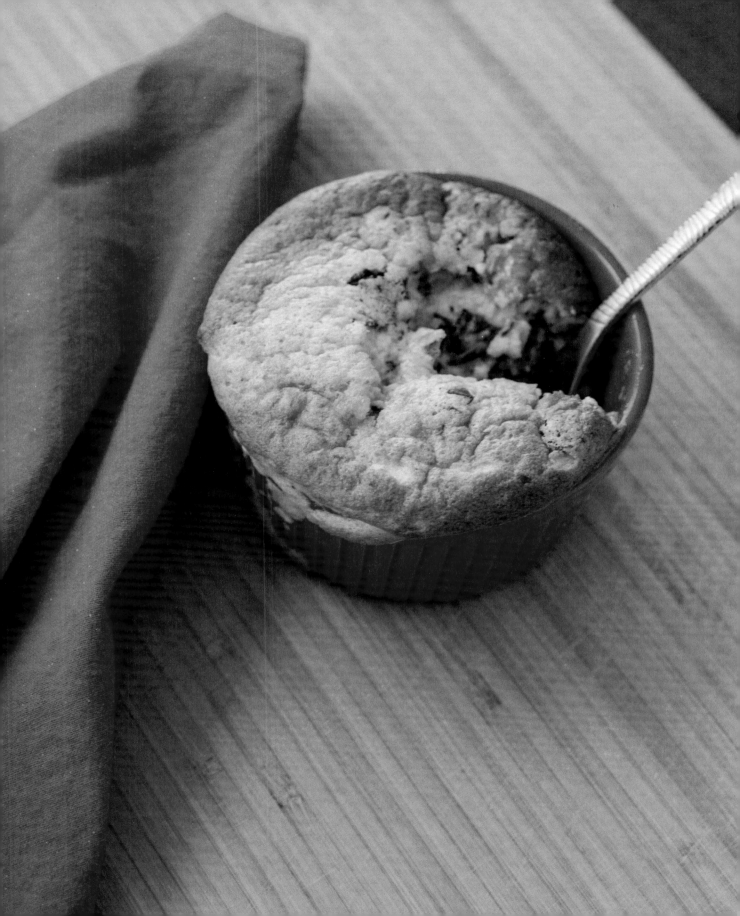

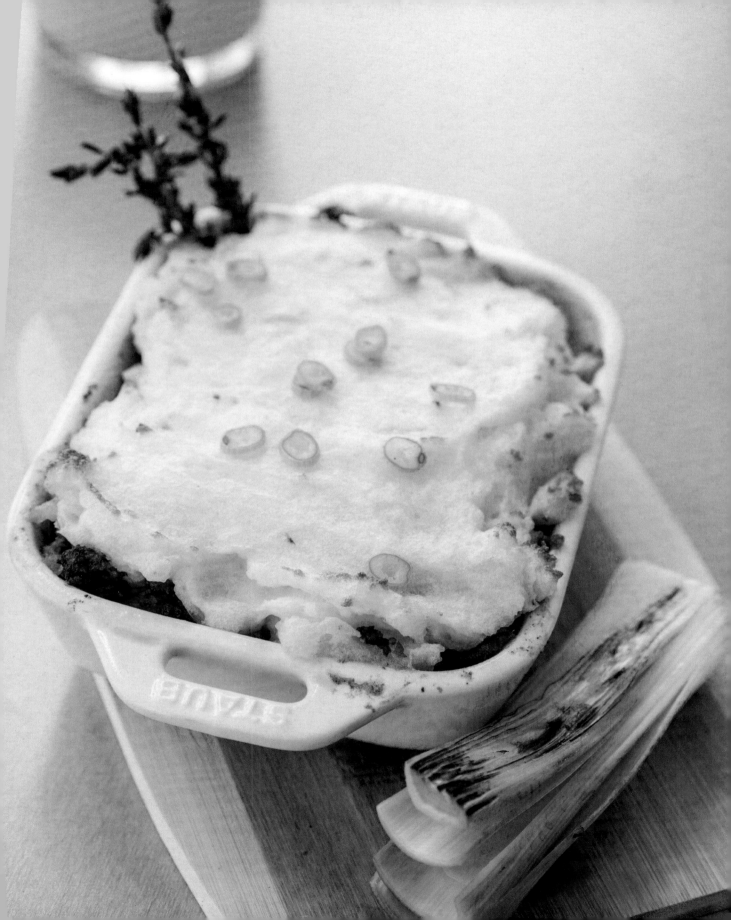

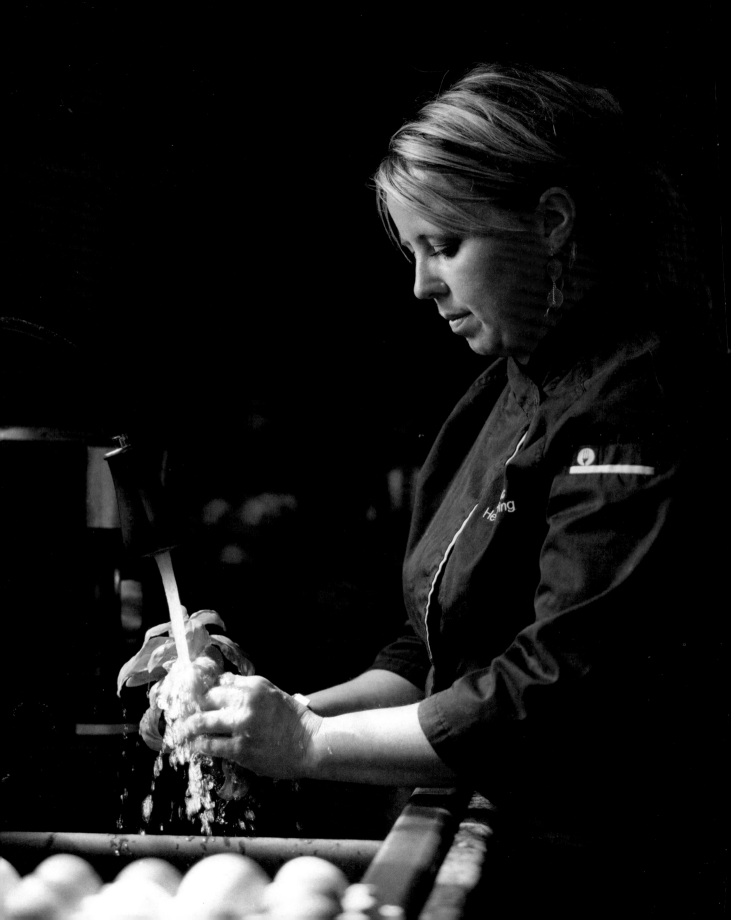